# At Home in a Nursing Home

**Life Course, Culture and Aging: Global Transformations**
*General Editor: Jay Sokolovsky, University of South Florida St. Petersburg*

Published by Berghahn Books under the auspices of the Association for Anthropology and Gerontology (AAGE) and the American Anthropological Association Interest Group on Aging and the Life Course.

The consequences of aging will influence most areas of contemporary life around the globe, from the makeup of households and communities and systems of care to attitudes toward health, disability and life's end. Engaging a cross-cultural framework, this series publishes monographs and collected works that examine these widespread transformations with a perspective on the entire life course and a particular focus on mid/late adulthood.

**Volume 9**
AT HOME IN A NURSING HOME
An Ethnography of Movement and Care in Australia
*Angela Rong Yang Zhang*

**Volume 8**
COLLABORATIVE HAPPINESS
Building the Good Life in Urban Cohousing Communities
*Catherine Kingfisher*

**Volume 7**
PREVENTING DEMENTIA?
Critical Perspectives on a New Paradigm of Preparing for Old Age
*Edited by Annette Leibing and Silke Schicktanz*

**Volume 6**
BEYOND FILIAL PIETY
Rethinking Aging and Caregiving in Contemporary East Asian Societies
*Edited by Jeanne Shea, Katrina Moore and Hong Zhang*

**Volume 5**
THE GLOBAL AGE-FRIENDLY COMMUNITY MOVEMENT
A Critical Appraisal
*Edited by Philip B. Stafford*

**Volume 4**
CARE ACROSS DISTANCE
Ethnographic Explorations of Aging and Migration
*Edited by Azra Hromadžić and Monika Palmberger*

**Volume 3**
AGING AND THE DIGITAL LIFE COURSE
*Edited by David Prendergast and Chiara Garattini*

**Volume 2**
UNFORGOTTEN
Love and the Culture of Dementia Care in India
*Bianca Brijnath*

**Volume 1**
TRANSITIONS AND TRANSFORMATIONS
Cultural Perspectives on Aging and the Life Course
*Edited by Caitrin Lynch and Jason Danely*

# AT HOME IN A NURSING HOME

## An Ethnography of Movement and Care in Australia

Angela Rong Yang Zhang

berghahn
NEW YORK • OXFORD
www.berghahnbooks.com

First published in 2023 by
Berghahn Books
www.berghahnbooks.com



**Library of Congress Cataloging-in-Publication Data**

Names: Zhang, Angela Rong Yang, author.
Title: At home in a nursing home : an ethnography of movement and care in Australia / Angela Rong Yang Zhang.
Description: New York : Berghahn Books, 2023. | Series: Life course, culture and aging: global transformations ; Volume 9 | Includes bibliographical references and index.
Identifiers: LCCN 2022019374 (print) | LCCN 2022019375 (ebook) | ISBN 9781800736641 (hardback) | ISBN 9781800736658 (ebook)
Subjects: LCSH: Older people--Nursing home care--Australia. | Nursing home care--Australia. | Older people--Services for--Australia.
Classification: LCC RA998.A8 Z43 2023 (print) | LCC RA998.A8 (ebook) | DDC 362.160994--dc23/eng/20220715
LC record available at https://lccn.loc.gov/2022019374
LC ebook record available at https://lccn.loc.gov/2022019375

**British Library Cataloguing in Publication Data**

A catalogue record for this book is available from the British Library

ISBN 978-1-80073-664-1 hardback
ISBN 978-1-80073-665-8 ebook

https://doi.org/10.3167/9781800736641

*For my dad, who suffered from Alzheimer's before he passed away, and my mum, a dedicated family carer who now lives in a nursing home, and finally, for my older self.*

# CONTENTS


List of Illustrations and Figures viii

Foreword
*Tim Ingold* x

Acknowledgements xiii

Prologue. Aged Care in Australia: Current Crisis and Context xvi

**Introduction.** Becoming at Home through Right Care 1

**Part I. Walking** 29

**1.** Watching Each Step 31

**2.** Beyond Wandering 46

**3.** Walking Out of the Freeze 60

**4.** Living in the Tension between Walking and Not Walking 72

**Part II. Care** 85

**5.** Care as Multiplicities 87

**6.** Caring at the Threshold of Life and Death 114

**Conclusion.** Becoming Ethical through Care 134

Epilogue 138

Afterword
*Philip B. Stafford* 139

Glossary 142

References 144

Index 152

# ILLUSTRATIONS AND FIGURES

## Illustrations


P.1. Deluxe bedroom. Image provided courtesy of Helpinghand. xxv

P.2. Deluxe private lounge. Image provided courtesy of Helpinghand. xxvi

P.3. A resident posing with an art and craft work of a dragon boat. The top left of the photograph shows part of the decoration, featuring the well-known Chinese painting 'Along the River during the Qingming Festival' of the Song dynasty. Image provided courtesy of Elder Chinese Home. xxvii

0.1. A resident interviewed in her room in the aged care facility in 2015. © Angela Zhang. 14

0.2. A resident and her cat in the aged care facility. Image provided courtesy of Elder Chinese Home. 15

0.3. Residents receiving visiting family and friends in the on-site café. Image provided courtesy of Helpinghand. 21

0.4. Outdoor café seating. Image provided courtesy of Helpinghand. 22

0.5. A hairdresser serving a resident in the on-site hair salon. Image provided courtesy of Helpinghand. 22

0.6. On-site chapel. Image provided courtesy of Helpinghand. 23

0.7. A resident gardening. Image provided courtesy of Helpinghand. 23

0.8. The ethnographer learning to walk with a walking frame and assistance from a physiotherapist in 2015. © Angela Zhang. 25

0.9. The ethnographer being assisted by two personal care workers with transferring from bed to chair in 2015. © Angela Zhang. 26

6.1. Dining area. Image provided courtesy of Helpinghand. 117

6.2. A resident posing with his birthday cake decorated using the Chinese character 'longevity'. Image provided courtesy of Elder Chinese Home. 120

## Figures

3.1. The 'roundabout' on the ground floor. The circle with a grey star in a black circle marks the seat in the middle of the roundabout; the square surrounding the circles marks the roundabout area; the arrows show people's walking routes towards the roundabout. Illustration: Michael Tianze Zhang. Published with permission. 61
3.2. Mr Harris' daily walking routine. The circle marks the seat in the middle of the roundabout; the grey star in a black circle marks Mr Harris' room; the arrows show Mr Harris' daily walking routes. Illustration: Michael Tianze Zhang. Published with permission. 62
4.1. Location of the lounge area and people's movements around it. The semi-circle with a grey star in a black circle marks the couches in the lounge area; the rectangle around it marks the lounge area; the arrows show people's movements around the lounge area. Illustration: Michael Tianze Zhang. Published with permission. 74

# FOREWORD

## Tim Ingold

TAKE A WALK IN THE woods, and you will encounter trees of all ages and sizes, from great veterans to diminutive saplings. The bark of ancient trees may be deeply furrowed, while knotty trunks attest to the violence wreaked by past storms. Some branches may have already succumbed to the ravages of time – dying off, if not already dead. Rot is setting in. Eventually, they will fall. Yet, for now, they still stand, if perhaps a little wonkily, their magnificence only enhanced by their singular and erratic appearance, spreading their boughs to provide genial cover for the undergrowth sprouting all around them. But then you come across a road leading to a clearing. Here, tucked away out of sight, is a scrapyard. It is populated by rusting and decrepit machines, from kitchen appliances to cars, whose parts no longer function and whose operators have long since left the scene. You cannot help comparing, in your mind, the respective fates of trees and machines, as they reach the end of life. And it came to my mind, too, as I read the beautiful book that is now in your hands.

The book is a study of what happens to old people in what are commonly called 'nursing homes'. These places have often been studied before, but rarely if ever with such clarity of insight into what it feels like for the real human beings who, for whatever reason, find themselves incarcerated within their walls. In terms of our analogy, these are people who once stood tall in the forest and were firmly rooted there. But now, with their roots cut, they are sequestered in the scrapyard. To be sure, if they have the means, the yard may be deluxe. It may be equipped with all possible comforts and conveniences and packed with electronics to monitor every conceivable variation in the condition of its inmates. But it is a scrapyard all the same. The bodies housed there, albeit of flesh and blood rather than metal and rubber, still malfunction. And like defunct machines, they once had intelligent operators to tell them what to do and direct their movements. But now these minds have gone missing, or are at least seriously impaired, leaving the bodies either inert and unresponsive or out of control.

It is of course a condition for all human beings, of any age, that they are present in the world, and alive to each other, only because they have, or rather *are*, bodies. The same goes for trees. But for humans as for trees, 'body' is really just shorthand for a plethora of movements and processes, like lines tightly bundled together but with loose ends trailing in every direction. For the tree, the trails are of roots below and shoots above; for people, they are of paths and tracks, threading through the ground. It is as such a bundle of trails that each of us comes into the world, at birth. Blossoming in life, this body-bundle becomes ever more entangled with other bodies around it. But as fast as some lines grow and proliferate, others shrivel and wither. Bodies age, and as they do, withering gradually outweighs proliferation. Barring sudden catastrophe, however, be it violent storm or fatal attack, body-bundles unravel only gradually. For people as for trees, life and death are not so much either/or conditions as concurrent processes. It can be hard to say exactly when one overtakes the other.

The metaphorical equivalence of humans and trees crops up in many languages and cultures. Even in English, we still speak of the trunk, limbs and crown of the body, and of our familial roots. We are also heirs, however, to another vision, which comes to us as a legacy of modern biomedicine and its more contemporary offshoot, cognitive neuroscience. In this vision, the body is likened to an exquisitely engineered machine, atop of which, in the driving seat, lies a central control unit, the mind-brain. The thing about the machine-body, as opposed to the tree-body, is that it is made up not of movements and processes but of moveable parts, joined up to form a totality that is complete in itself. Far from tangling with its environs, such a body inserts itself in between, both separating mind from world and mediating the action of one upon the other. Once it wears out and can be of no further service, it is sent as scrap for decommissioning. And at the heart of this book is the clash of metaphors in a society that treats the human equivalent of its old-growth forest as a scrapyard.

In the forest, trees grow older together. Their lives are intertwined, both below and above ground. Is this not equally true of human beings? People, too, endlessly create themselves, and one another, in the crucible of their common life. It is from the matrix of their relations with others, and with everything else in their surroundings that matters to them, that they draw the power of renewal. Colloquially, we call this matrix 'home'. Just what it means to make a place a home is a central theme of this book. The theme revolves around two related keywords, namely 'care' and 'habit'. The home is a place of habitation, and it is also a place of care. These words have in common that they fall foul of the distinction, so often taken for granted, between active and passive voices of the verb, or between doing and being done to. Do we make our habits, we wonder, or do our habits make us? Do we care, or are we cared for? The real answer, surely, is neither or both of the above. For just as habitation makes the inhabitant, caring creates the carer.

So long as we remain standing in the forest, we are not forced to take sides. Nor need we do so at home. In the intertwining of lives, be they of trees or people, caring is also being cared *for*. The old continue to care for the young, all the more so in the latter's caring for them. After all, in joining hands, who is to say which hand holds and which is held? To care and be cared for is not to be on one side or the other but to be literally in the midst. Home, here, is a *milieu*, literally a middle place. In the space of bodily decommissioning, however, all that changes. For in the deluxe scrapyard that is the 'nursing home', care takes on the nature of a transaction. On one side are providers of care, in full possession of their cognitive faculties. On the other side are recipients, whose faculties have partially or wholly deserted them. The first do the caring; the second have care done to them. In between are malfunctioning bodily machines. All at once, the very idea of 'home' is cleft in twain.

Not only care is split. So too are such basic functions as walking, sitting and eating. With this, the restless stirrings of the soul are deemed an agitation that calls for physical restraint, lest it gets out of hand or leads to falls, and the joy of commensality is recast as a dietary regime to be administered. Elderly residents do not walk, sit and eat but are walked, sat and fed. This book tells movingly of the tragic consequences of this split, along with the efforts of both staff and residents to avert it, ever frustrated by a culture of managerialism in hock to biomedical discourses. Yet the book leaves us uplifted rather than depressed, for two reasons. First, we find that old people whose minds may be at a loss, and who seem to those who know them to be but shadows of their former selves, can nevertheless – given the chance – find joy and beauty in the world beyond the comprehension of those of us still wrapped in our quotidian lives. And the second lies in showing a better way to look after our old people. It is to abandon the scrapyard and return to the forest!

Aberdeen, January 2022

**Tim Ingold** is Professor Emeritus of Social Anthropology at the University of Aberdeen. He has carried out fieldwork among Saami and Finnish people in Lapland, and has written on environment, technology and social organization in the circumpolar North, on animals in human society, and on human ecology and evolutionary theory. His more recent work explores environmental perception and skilled practice. Ingold's current interests lie on the interface between anthropology, archaeology, art and architecture. His recent books include *The Perception of the Environment* (2000), *Lines* (2007), *Being Alive* (2011), *Making* (2013), *The Life of Lines* (2015), *Anthropology and/as Education* (2018) and *Anthropology: Why it Matters* (2018). He is also the editor, inter alia, of *Companion Encyclopedia of Anthropology* (1994).

# ACKNOWLEDGEMENTS

WRITING A BOOK IS LIKE walking a path or weaving many lives, events, objects and ideas together in meaningful ways. This book involves the contributions of many people. Of course, the book would not have been possible at all without the participation of the elderly people whom I met during my fieldwork in the nursing homes. Thank you all for allowing me the opportunity to walk alongside you, and for teaching me about your ways of feeling and thinking about home and care in the nursing homes.

Doing fieldwork in a care home was harder than I thought and more rewarding than I could have imagined. I remain profoundly grateful to the staff members who welcomed me in the aged care facilities. Your dedication, compassion and insights inspired my exploration of right care and helped me to see alternative approaches for care provision. To the management team in two residential facilities, I thank you for giving your permission and providing support to this project. I am also grateful to the many people, including family and friends of residents, volunteers, visiting health and allied health professionals, who talked to me and supported this project in various ways.

Guiding me along this path and teaching me their crafts were my academic mentors, Professor John Gray and Dr Tanya Zivkovic, to whom I extend my deepest gratitude; they have been fundamental in the creation of this book. Professor John Gray supported this project from its inception and pointed me towards the phenomenologically oriented anthropological approach, which turned out to be fruitful. I'm extremely grateful to Dr Tanya Zivkovic for her mentorship and for always encouraging me to explore and improve my work. Without her patient guidance, I couldn't have seen this project through. I'm eternally grateful to them both for their guidance at every step of this project. I thank them for their ongoing support, shrewd criticism and seasoned advice.

Very special thanks go to Professor Megan Warin. Your insightful comments on my work led me to see the intrinsic connections between home, movement and care, which helped me to build a coherent structure for this book. To Professor Simone Dennis, I thank you, too, for pointing me to the notion of power, and how power infiltrates care. Also to Dr Rod Lucas, I thank you for your support at the early stage of this project.

To Professor Tim Ingold, I owe you a special debt of gratitude. My wildest dreams came true when you responded to my email and agreed to write a foreword for this book. Thank you, Professor. Your writings on movement and walking opened my eyes and my mind and lit a pathway into the hidden dimensions of the lived realities of ageing and aged care.

To Dr Philip Stafford, I am very grateful to you for contributing an afterword to this book. Your edited book, *Gray Areas: Ethnographic Encounters with Nursing Home Culture*, was my traveller's guidebook as I walked the process of this project.

Although this path into the field of academia has not always been a smooth ride, I treasure my time at the University of Adelaide, Department of Anthropology and Development Studies. To academic and professional staff in the Department and School of Social Sciences: Dr Susan Hemer, Associate Professor Georgina Drew, Dr Alison Dundun, Dr Dianne Rodger, Professor Andrew Skuse, Professor Melissa Jane Nursey-Bray, Ms Shamira Barr, Dr Anna Szorenyi and Associate Professor Russell Brewer, I thank you for lending your support to this project and its publication. To Dr William Skinner and Dr Gail Wright, I also thank you for your comments on my work at the disciplinary seminars.

Bringing a book to life is akin to opening up a field in which different ways of living, moving and thinking meet, connect and correspond. I would like to pay my special regards to Associate Editor Tom Bonnington. Thank you, Tom, for being patient and supportive. It is because of your advice and encouragement that this book has been moulded into its current shape. To Production Editor Dr Caroline Kuhtz and everyone on the Berghahn Books publishing team, I thank you for your work and for guiding me through the production process.

I would also like to thank two anonymous reviewers for their helpful comments that improved the manuscript.

To Valerie Mobley, I'm forever indebted to your invaluable contribution, not only in editing and proofreading the manuscript but also in sharing your comments, ideas and experiences with aged care facilities as a family member of residents. I would also like to thank Sarah Sibley for copyediting the manuscript.

To Megan Davis, Minerva Lau and Kevin Poon, I'd like to express my gratitude for your permission to include the photographs in the book, which allow readers a visual glimpse into the nursing home environments. To Yu Qiao and Cindy Luo, I thank you for your contribution to the engaging cover image. Especially, I would like to thank Michael Tianze Zhang for creating the illustrations of residents walking and sitting. To Dr Kathy

Radoslovich, I am very grateful for your kind help in securing my access into facilities for my fieldwork.

I must also thank Donald Dong Zhang for indexing work and technical support. Whenever I had a problem, you always came to the rescue using your computer skills.

To Yaping Zhou, Maureen Simmonds, Megan Cho, Mahima Light, Jinxia Cui and Lixin Wang, I learned from your experiences and insights; I appreciate your unfailing support for my work. Thanks go to others who have played a part in this journey: Jan Van Emden, Marta Skibicki, Julie Kahl, Albert Lee, Sandy Liew, Di Fuamoli, Jessica Noakes, Sharon Neighbour, Dr Jayne Curnow, Dr Deane Fergie, Helen Attar, Sharon Lewis, Helen Nagel and John Liddle.

Finally. To Mum: you are my source of inspiration. Your love and support for me never waver.

# PROLOGUE
# AGED CARE IN AUSTRALIA
## Current Crisis and Context

### Aged Care in Crisis

In early 2017, an investigation into the death of Mr Bob Spriggs, a former resident of the Makk and McLeay Nursing Home at the Oakden Aged Mental Health Care Service, operated by the South Australian government's Department of Health, revealed some concerning practices in the facility. Mr Spriggs was reported to have been subjected to significant chemical and physical restraints. In the final weeks of his life, he was overdosed with 10 times his prescribed amount of antipsychotic medication on at least three occasions. He also had bruises thought to be caused from being restrained in a chair.

Intriguingly, the use of restraints was identified by the South Australian chief psychiatrist as a routine workplace practice (Groves et al. 2017). Staff at the Oakden facility considered restraint to be the only effective measure to stop residents attempting to stand or to walk, and thus reduce their risk of fall-related injuries. Before its closure in April 2017, the Makk and McLeay Nursing Home had provided long-term subsidized residential aged care to older people with severe or extreme behavioural problems or, to use the medical term, behavioural and psychological symptoms of dementia (BPSD). Mr Spriggs had Parkinson's disease and Lewy body dementia. His admission to the Makk and McLeay Nursing Home was due to his extreme BPSD.

Drawing on a medical model of managing BPSD (Brodaty, Draper and Low 2003) and evidence showing the facility's failure to use an appropriate model of care, a Senate inquiry into the Oakden facility concluded that the care provided there was 'not the right care' for the residents (The Senate Community Affairs Committee Secretariat 2018: 30). Here, 'right care' is considered within the logic of dementia diagnosis to be the correct use of a suitable model to manage symptoms that are thought to be harmful to patients themselves and people around them.

Doing fieldwork in two aged care homes in Adelaide, South Australia during the time that the Oakden facility was under investigation, I had the opportunity to learn about 'right care', not from health experts or policymakers but from nursing home residents themselves, including some who had dementia and BPSD. I witnessed how aged and frail residents felt an urge to move, made efforts to put one foot in front of the other, and depended on the assistance of other supportive people and things to move safely. In contrast to the biomedical construct of BPSD, which was often deployed as a rationale to restrain bodies, it was in doing the most mundane activities of walking, moving and eating that residents could experience an expansion of their social and relational lifeworlds beyond their individual bodily constraints and ailments.

However, reduced funding and limited access to staff assistance meant residents could sometimes be confined to chairs to prevent them from walking unaided and having falls. I came to understand how moving, or not moving, revealed the politics of care. When residents' calls for help and efforts to move are treated as symptoms, and their bodies managed through practices of restraint, whose concerns are being taken care of? As this book will show, what counts as 'care' in the current aged care system in Australia favours the concerns of governments and providers and neglects the immediate bodily experience of people who receive care.

A current failure to understand of life as it is lived in and through the aged body is highly consequential. While numerous ethical, political, biomedical, economic and other deliberations attend to the residential aged care sector, only certain kinds of questions are asked and answered about the *quality of care* and how to supply it. In challenging the prevailing emphasis on how the aged care sector could be improved financially, clinically and infrastructurally, I propose to think instead about how to deliver aged care *with care*: to examine the complexity of the lived realities of ageing, to decipher what it means 'to care', and to engage with viewpoints that have been neglected.

This book asks how older people could be enabled to move and to live a good life in a nursing home. In doing so, it seeks to trouble the thinking that has been partly responsible for the aged care crisis in Australia and to signal an alternative approach to manage the bodily realities of ageing and the bureaucracy of aged care provision. As I will argue in this book, care needs to be delivered in a way that is responsive to residents' bodies, to their desires and efforts to move, despite the constraints imposed by an increasingly standardized and commoditized aged care sector.

We cannot but care. Caring is not an option but a vital necessity, as ageing will affect all of us and our families in various ways. The question of how to make care right for people receiving care pleads for our attention. In the search for answers, I will place this study of nursing homes into a local context. But first I want to trace the historical origins of the nursing home in Australia and its contemporary fashioning into the aged care facility. In so doing, I will highlight the forces, ideologies, discourses and concerns of governments and providers that have fashioned the aged care system in Australia today.

## The Context: From Nursing Home to Residential Aged Care

### *Nursing Home: What Is in the Name?*

During my visit to one facility, I was told by the manager that the term ‘nursing home’ is no longer used today. ‘This is the first thing to learn if you want to research aged care,’ she said. This change in nomenclature is just one part of a shift in thinking about how residential aged care should be designed, funded and packaged to suit an ageing demographic. Many things, according to the manager, had changed for the better, including the name. ‘Nowadays, we call this place a residential aged care facility,’ she said. I wanted to understand why the term ‘residential aged care facility’ is now preferred over ‘nursing home’; what had changed over time, and how might these changes have contributed (or not) to residents’ experiences and adjustments when entering residential care? But even before I could raise my questions, she began telling me how she started working as a carer in this very same facility, more than thirty years ago.

> You wouldn’t believe what a nursing home was like back then. Six people shared one big room. There were only curtains to provide the residents with some privacy. When we attended to one resident, everyone else could hear what was going on. It was awful. Now, all the residents’ rooms are single-bedded, or double-bedded for couples. The whole facility is newly renovated and uplifted to make it look more spacious, bright and cheerful. Although the residents are older, sicker and more fragile, the aiding equipment we have now, such as lifters, wheelchairs and hospital beds, makes the work so much easier. Back in the old days, working as a carer was heavy physical work. I almost broke my back!

This account spoke to a shared view that the term ‘nursing home’ no longer represents what the facility is and certainly does not describe the people who live there or work there. Accordingly, that term is no longer used in contemporary aged care policy and practice. Nowadays, the organization delivering care for elderly people is known as an ‘aged care service provider’, and the physical setting providing accommodation and care for the aged is a ‘residential aged care facility’. However, in the field, I noticed that residents, family members and care staff routinely used the terms 'nursing home' and 'nursing home residents'; and so, wishing to use the language actually used by my study participants, I also use those terms in this book. But even as I do so, I reflect on the multiple and contested meanings of the idea of the nursing home – the names that have come to define and redefine it, and the underlying thinking of those who design policy and those who enact it. In this chapter, I will seek to trace the making and the unmaking of the nursing home over time as I examine the associated diverse forces at play, including government funding schemes, social ideologies of medicine and economy, and multiple bureaucratic processes that guide daily practices. My aim is to provide a social, political and historical context for this book's fundamental question of how residents come to feel at home in nursing homes through right care. I will start by tracing the evolution of institutional care for the aged in Australia.

### *Contested Cultural Space*

The very expression 'nursing home' reflects the contested ideas and practices entangled in our concept of institutional care for the aged. While we associate the concept of 'home' with private property, independent living, domesticity and family relationships, 'nursing', by contrast, evokes more clinical associations. This seeming contradiction and ambiguity in the term itself was captured by US anthropologist Philip Stafford in his introduction to a collection of ethnographic nursing home studies, *Gray Areas: Ethnographic Encounters with Nursing Home Culture*. Stafford attributes the collective discomfort with the term to its 'ambiguous status in the cultural order, owing to its being composed of elements drawn from oppositional spheres of meaning: home and hospital', which renders it, he says, a 'contested cultural space' (2003a: 10). In this study of the Australian context, we see that the contestation goes beyond the imperatives of medicine and domesticity to include the combined forces of public government funding and capital investment from the private sector. Over time, the interplay of these forces has led to the increased complexity that has rendered not only the name but the very purpose of the nursing home ambiguous.

### *Home for the Homeless and Aged: Funding Care*

Prior to 1900 in Australia, assistance from benevolent charities was the primary means of relief for people who could not support themselves (ABS 1988). The benevolent asylums (called the 'Destitute Asylum' in South Australia) were institutions established throughout the colonies of Australia in the nineteenth century to house the homeless. Victoria had nine benevolent asylums in 1857 (Hull et al. 1863), while in 1860, there were eleven benevolent asylums in New South Wales (The Sydney Morning Herald 1860). The Destitute Asylum in Adelaide, South Australia was established in 1851 (George and George 2011). The inmates were not predominantly old people. Asylums took in anyone who was poor, destitute, disabled or aged, and many focused on care for children and pregnant women.

As the population aged, the needs of older people (mostly men) who were ill and destitute were increasingly recognized. The Melbourne Benevolent Asylum was built in 1851 (Kehoe 1998) as a social institution for the aged and sick. At the time of its origin, it stood at the periphery of society, mostly developed through Christian charitable organizations and financed by government grants and charity money. In its early years, the Melbourne Benevolent Asylum was 'filled to repletion with aged and infirm persons, many of them labouring under complicated diseases' (Whitehead 2018). More benevolent asylums were built in the following years in Melbourne. These institutions received maintenance subsidies for pensioners from 1909 to 1963 and provided disadvantaged residents with basic shelter and meals.

During the Second World War, an Australian Labor government, seeking to create a welfare state, enacted a series of national schemes for unemployment, sickness and special benefits for the socioeconomically disadvantaged (ABS 1988). The nursing home as we know it became a mainstream and federally funded social welfare institution when the federal government stepped into the aged care field in 1954 with the *Aged Person's Homes Act*. The Act provided subsidies to approved charitable organizations to provide essentially self-contained hostel accommodation. Most of the rapid growth in the number of nursing home beds occurred between 1962 and 1972, following the introduction, by the Menzies government, of a 20 shillings ($2) per day per resident nursing home benefit in approved nursing homes (Guen 1993). The private sector was quick to seize the opportunity to move in for profit. In the five years between 1963 and 1968, the number of new nursing homes grew by 20 per cent, and the number of beds added to existing homes grew by 48 per cent (Parker 1987: 14). In 1982, the residential aged care sector provided some 140 beds for every 1,000 Australians aged over 75 years – one of the highest ratios of beds to people in the world (Guen 1993: 1). However, with its undesirable association with old age and impending death, going into nursing home accommodation was seen as a last resort for old and sick people. Certainly, as the facility manager described it to me, nursing homes back then were nothing like the domestic haven that the word 'home' suggests today.

The status of the nursing home as a social welfare institution has been regularly re-examined because of the changing socioeconomic situation of the country, as well as its demographic of ageing citizens. The problem of shortage of accommodation for the aged in the early 1940s looked very different by the early 1970s, when the McMahon government presided over uncontrolled growth of private nursing home accommodation, accompanied by a rapid increase of government spending on nursing home subsidies (Guen 1993: 4). One solution to this burgeoning cost was to support those elderly people who were socioeconomically disadvantaged, rather than wealthier retired taxpayers and owners of private homes.

For the poor and disadvantaged, special supplements, as specified in Section 11-3 of the *Aged Care Act 1997*, were put in place. These included: a homeless supplement, to support aged care homes caring for people with a history of, or who were at risk of homelessness; a hardship supplement, paid to support recipients suffering financial hardship; and an accommodation supplement for those unable to pay all or part of their accommodation costs. With the provision of shelter through a range of public housing measures (such as through the South Australian Housing Trust), a change of focus from 'housing' to 'care' emerged, and the moving from home into a nursing home was deemed unnecessary if an older person was not in need of nursing care. Thus, instead of being supported accommodation for the homeless and aged, the nursing home became increasingly a place of nursing practice, reflecting a pivotal shift in federal government aged care policy and funding.

With the coming of the Hawke Labor government in 1983, the notion of a nursing home as a bounded physical site gradually dissolved because of the ongoing reforms of aged care government funding policy (Guen 1993: 4). Under the policy of 'ageing in place in aged care', introduced in the late 1990s, hostel beds providing low-level care, and nursing home beds providing high-level care were offered within the one facility so that residents could move seamlessly from one to the other as they became frailer (AIHW 2002). Furthermore, instead of the term 'nursing home bed' in aged care policy, the more abstract 'nursing home place' was constructed, which referred to a status of eligibility for government-funded care in a residential facility. Instead of referring to a concrete, physical and bounded residential setting in which the aged would be accommodated and cared for, the term 'nursing home' increasingly became associated with federal government aged care funding and resource distribution.

Alongside the abstract constructions of 'nursing home place' and 'nursing home bed', the term 'nursing home care' appeared in the context of policy changes that placed a new emphasis on the provision of nursing practice. Before the 2012 aged care reform,[1] the term 'nursing home' primarily referred to high-level care and the residential setting where this type of care was provided. One of the aims of the reform was to move towards providing more support and care for the elderly at home.

### *High (Nursing Home) Care: Medicalizing Needs*

The construction of 'nursing home place' in policy and funding schemes sought to differentiate those older Australians who were considered in need of nursing care from those who were not. Only those assessed as in need of care and eligible to take up a nursing home place could be admitted into residential aged care facilities. The medicalization of needs and care was evident in this process of differentiation. In Australia, one crucial step to medicalize the arena of aged care was the introduction of the aged care assessment in 1972. The approval of a medical practitioner was required prior to an older person's admission to a nursing home, which was also required to be endorsed (or rejected) by a federal medical officer (Guen 1993: 14). The Australian Government then announced in August 1986 that a comprehensive health assessment was necessary to help older persons avoid unnecessary nursing home admission. The assessment was made by teams of specialists who became known as geriatric assessment teams. The name was changed to aged care assessment team (ACAT) in 1992 because many older people objected to the negative connotations now associated with the term geriatric (Guen 1993: 5–14).

Eligibility assessment was the initial step in the medicalization of the social welfare sector of aged care. Both the welfare state and its ageing citizens as nursing home residents are now defined through the practice of medicalized assessments of care needs. As part and parcel of the 'medicalization of old age and death' (Kearl 1996: 340), medicine dominates in the arena of aged care, especially in the residential care settings. Stafford (2003a) suggests that the nursing home is primarily a medical institution in which the ideology of medicine, as a set of organized ideas, is in full play. As 'the individual patient's "problem" is seen as a health problem (disease) that needs treatment' (Stafford 2003a: 6), nursing home residents are categorized and understood through their diseases. In the 2012 report of the Australian Institute of Health and Welfare (AIHW 2012), residents are represented using disease categories and incidence rates, such as circulatory system diseases (24%), diseases of the musculoskeletal system and connective tissue (18%), endocrine, nutritional and metabolic disorders (8%) and cognitive impairment with dementia (52%). Eligibility assessment focuses on the presence or absence of disease and extent of pathology, which defines who can or cannot access nursing home care and residential accommodation. In turn, ongoing care level assessments determine the availability of aiding devices and equipment to residents, as well as facility funding levels.

### *Aged Care as Industry: Commoditizing Care*

Under the accumulative pressure of government budget deficit, the once heavily government-subsidized aged care system evolved into a profitable service industry in Australia, as it did in other developed Western countries.[2] In Australia, the co-contribution funding model, launched as part of the 2012 aged care reform, further accelerated the process of commercialization in this business-oriented sector. In the context of policy and industry, residential aged care refers to a type of commoditized service, providing accommodation, everyday living support (meals, laundry and cleaning), nursing and personal care services. It is subsidized by the Australian Government, offered by a service provider and partly paid for by residents and their families. The services categorized as 'care' are central in residential aged care. It is the element of care that gives the name, shape and form to this sector. While everyday living support with meals, cleaning and laundry are provided under the category of housekeeping and itemized separately, they are essential to the daily delivery of care.

The word 'care' is used in this context of 'care practice' to refer to the organized activities aimed at maintaining a liveable everyday life for older people. There are two main types of care practice in a residential setting: nursing care and personal care. Nursing care (or 'health care' as it has been called more recently), including medication management, continence and catheter care and wound treatment, is available to residents 24/7 from qualified nursing staff. 'Personal care services' include varying levels of assistance with bathing, toileting, eating, dressing, mobility and managing incontinence (Productivity Commission 2011a: 25). Personal care is mostly delivered in the form of assisting residents with their activities of daily living (ADLs), which is a term now regularly used in the sector.

There is a hierarchy of work in nursing homes, with the 'dirty' personal care work at the bottom – namely, cleaning body waste, showering and toileting – and the 'clean' office paperwork at the top. Nursing care and personal care are delivered by different staff – staff with different qualifications and positioned differently in the institutional hierarchy. While care staff spend most of their shift time engaging intimately with residents, doing the hands-on care activities, others – nursing, medical and allied health professionals – often spend most of their working hours doing paperwork. There is a hierarchy of status in nursing home staff, corresponding to the type of work involved. As is widely acknowledged in the aged care system, the more educated and trained the staff, the higher their rank will be and the further away they will be from daily care practices for the residents. The institutional power is always initiated from the top of the hierarchy, the 'office', where the executives and administrators conduct their daily work, down to the bottom of the hierarchy, the 'floor', where the residents live and daily care work is carried out. Contrary to the imagery of customer-centricity that aged care providers strive to create, residents are positioned 'at the bottom layer', as care workers said, of the power structure.

Organized staff assistance permeates the everyday lives of nursing home residents and often gives the care facility its institutional look and feel. Based on covert ethnographic research undertaken as a certified nursing assistant or 'nursing aide' (or, in Australian terminology, a 'personal care worker') in three different nursing homes, Timothy Diamond's (1992) *Making Gray Gold: Narratives of Nursing Home Care*, offers an insider's view and interpretation of nursing home life. He places the nursing aides' hands-on caregiving activities and the institutional recording of that activity, the text, at the centre of his analysis, showing how daily care practice is structured by institutionally prescribed and documented tasks, such as the two-hourly repositioning of bedridden residents. His observations reveal a parallel existence: the lived realities of residents and nursing aides, and the institutional structures imposed by the quasi-capitalist labour and service system that governs the nursing homes. The assertion that an economic imperative lies at the heart of nursing home operations is confirmed by other research that found that the organization of work in nursing homes is geared towards getting work done with the maximum economy of human resources (Bland 2007: 942).

In recent years, in response to the demands of the more prosperous generation of 'baby boomers', now retiring, there have been more changes to the residential aged care industry. There is now another measure, the Extra Service status, which enables service providers to charge more for higher standards of accommodation (Department of Health and Ageing 2012b: 43). One Adelaide care facility, Dulce Domum, underwent extensive renovations after a change of ownership brought additional investment and it became affiliated to a large multistate aged care service provider. All its beds were approved by the government for Extra Service status, and the service provider advertised the facility on its corporate website as 'a major investment' that offers 'genuine value for money'.

The new fee structure provides more flexibility in a business model for residential aged care and allows the sector to become more market-led and competitive. Older persons and their families now become customers, and in accordance with a neoliberal policy agenda, they are now given more choice about what services they want and how much they are willing to pay for them. Driven by growing competition in a customer-centric market, it becomes a strategic priority to remodel and renovate aged care facilities in order to attract affluent residents by gauging and meeting their preferences. Nursing home facilities can thus be upgraded to attract clients who can pay additional fees for better amenities and services, be they elderly people themselves or families who want to pay extra for premium accommodation.

The website of Auxilia, a not-for-profit aged care provider, describes what their 'extra services' might look like in tempting promotional copy. Residents could be offered suites, rather than single rooms – that is, a separate bedroom (see Illustration P.1) and lounge (see Illustration P.2). Single rooms could be a spacious 16m$^2$ in size, with an ensuite bathroom. These rooms, described as 'premium rooms', are 'beautifully appointed, with designer-selected superior décor and fittings ... and overlook gardens, the courtyard, or attractive views'. Along with such superior accommodation, potential residents are able to access a range of included services, such as hairdressing, beauty treatments, daily newspapers and à la carte 3-course menus.

Extra Service status allows providers to charge more money through the 'extra services agreement'. In return, they will provide 'hotel-type services, such as better accommodation, food and services' to residents who enter aged care under this agreement (Department of Health 2020). With elements akin to luxury hotels, such as a grand lobby, refined interior decoration, 'deluxe' private suites, and an emphasis on the etiquette and manners of staff, the commoditization of care is increasingly evident in the residential aged care sector in Australia. However, for many Australians, moving into a nursing home is financially unfeasible. For people who have

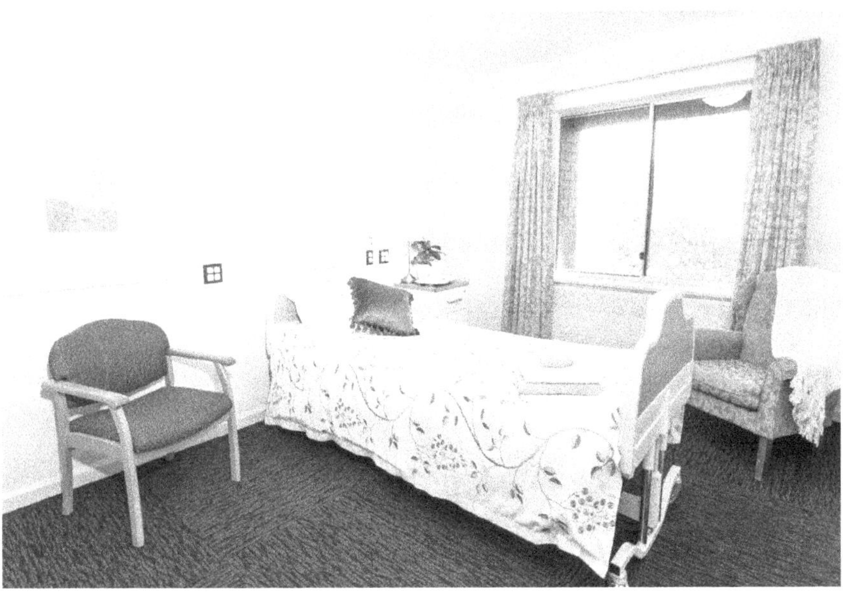

**ILLUSTRATION P.1.** Deluxe bedroom. Image provided courtesy of Helpinghand.

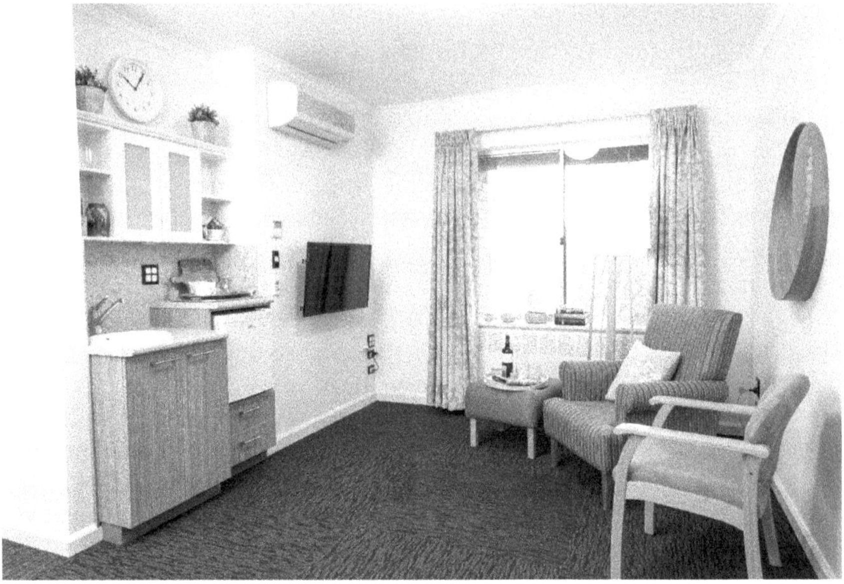

ILLUSTRATION P.2. Deluxe private lounge. Image provided courtesy of Helpinghand.

no or limited assets and need financial hardship assistance to enter residential aged care, their options may be limited to low-cost facilities where the 'standard' accommodation can be a world away from Extra Services.

## Home-Like Environment: Domesticizing Everyday Experience

In her ethnographic study set in two Australian residential aged care facilities, Fiveash (1998) reveals the uncomfortable experiences of residents that stem from the public nature of nursing home living. As one of her participants said, 'I have no private place of my own' (Fiveash 1998: 169). Much of the distress recounted by residents in her study arose from the involuntary sharing of rooms and spaces (Fiveash 1998: 168). This echoes the facility manager's remarks that I quoted at the beginning of this chapter, pointing out that the crowded nursing homes of the past stood in stark contrast to the residential aged care facility of today.

With the word 'home' replaced by the more clinically oriented term 'facility', service providers are often impelled by an imagined cultural conception of 'home' to create a home-like appearance and ambience in their facilities (See Illustration P.3). In a care facility I visited in Melbourne, which provides specialized care for elderly Australians from a Chinese cultural

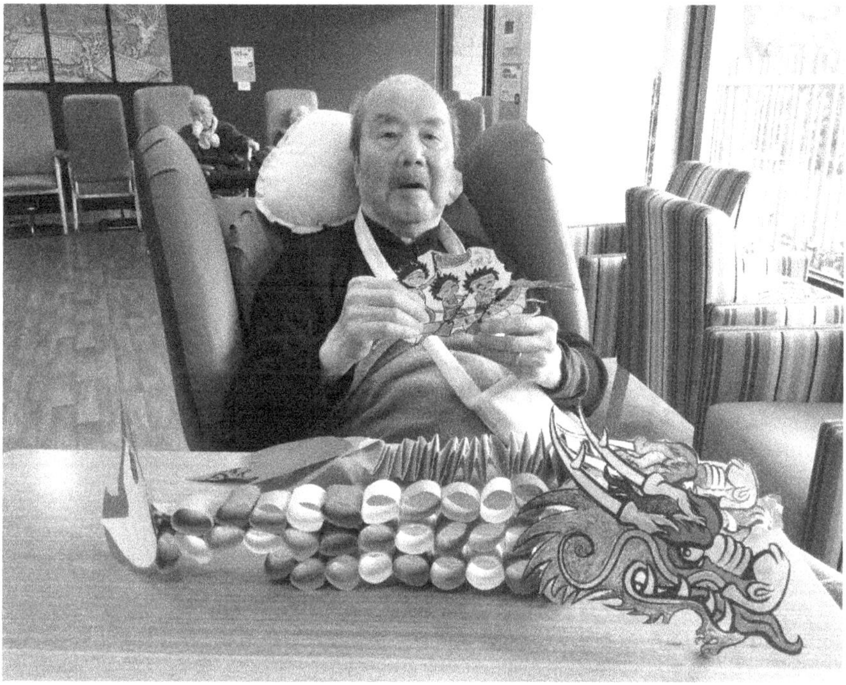

**ILLUSTRATION P.3.** A resident posing with an art and craft work of a dragon boat. The top left of the photograph shows part of the decoration, featuring the well-known Chinese painting 'Along the River during the Qingming Festival' of the Song dynasty. Image provided courtesy of Elder Chinese Home.

background, Chinese cultural elements such as the statue of Maitreya (also known as the Big Belly or Laughing Buddha) and the poster with the upside-down Chinese character 'Fu' (a pun indicating the befalling of happiness) prominently decorate residents' lounges and doors.

In their aim to create a home-like physical environment through architectural features, interior decor and personalized bedrooms, service providers seek to provide residents with their own space in which to feel comfortable and at ease. However, given the public nature of nursing home living, these environmental modifications may amount to a quite superficial presentation of what home might look or feel like. Indeed, as I will show in this book, 'some institutions have taken on the trappings [of home] ... without fundamentally questioning the presumptions of care and basic human needs' (Stafford 2003a: 20).

The history of residential aged care and changing socioeconomic pressures in Australia have combined to produce the material realities of today's nursing homes. Although these multiple ideologies, discourses, concerns and practices shape how people will live out their final years, none of these components can provide an answer to how an elderly resident might come to feel at home in a nursing home. Home, as this book will show, is more than physical objects, persons, living environments or practices. I argue that aged care residents experience 'home' as a sense of 'rightness' of being that comes from the intertwining of multiple things and people that assist them to do the things that they want to do but are unable to do independently. In the next chapter, I will introduce my own ethnographic study and invite readers to join me in the residential facilities that formed the setting for this study. I will introduce the analytical lens of 'right care' and 'becoming-at-home' that I chose as the theoretical framework for the study and will explain the vital importance of movement in achieving 'right care'.

## Notes

1. The 2012 aged care reform, also referred to as the Living Longer Living Better reforms, was announced by the Gillard federal Labor government in response to the *Caring for Older Australians* report, prepared by the Productivity Commission in 2011.
2. Importantly, population ageing is an international issue that has led to increased care needs for the elderly in many non-Western countries, as well. One prominent example is China, which has seen significant growth in the aged care industry. By 2018, as reported in Xinhua, a Chinese state-run news source, China had 28,000 registered nursing institutes for the elderly and more than seven million elderly nursing home beds (https://gbtimes.com/china-has-28000-registered-nursing-homes, viewed on 15 April 2020).

# INTRODUCTION

## Becoming at Home through Right Care

### 'At Home' in Old Age

'I want to go home', Mr Harris sighed as he held on to his walker, hauled himself upright, and walked away. Mr Harris lived in the aged care facility where I undertook fieldwork, and we spent many an hour and day walking together. Sitting opposite the main entrance of the facility, Mr Harris would routinely fix his gaze at the glass doors, through which people constantly came and went. Every resident leaving the facility had to be accompanied by someone, a staff member, a relative or friend, a volunteer or visitor, who would unlock the door by entering a security code – a string of characters printed in tiny font on a notice affixed to the wall next to the security lock. Added was a reminder: 'Close the door behind you to prevent the residents from absconding.' With a grave look, Mr Harris whispered to me, 'This is imprisonment.' He then added that he intended to ask his daughter to get him out of this place the next time she came to visit.

A few days after my chat with Mr Harris, I discovered that he was 'out' as he had wished – his daughter had taken him on 'social leave' to spend the weekend with her family. I felt happy for him – he could have a break from routinized nursing home life and spend time with his family. However, in the late afternoon, and to everyone's surprise, Mr Harris was back inside the facility in time for afternoon tea. Distraught and exhausted, his daughter explained the situation to me. After a car trip to the beach and a fun picnic, the family had returned home. Mr Harris then became restless, walking all over the house looking for his own room. When she told her father that he would be spending the night in her spare bedroom, he grew more distressed and insisted that he should return before it got too late. So, feeling confused and heartbroken, his daughter took him back to the facility. After joining other residents in the dining area for some soup and bread, Mr Harris looked his usual self. Pushing his red 4-wheeled walker, he was back on his feet, walking again.

How can we understand the perplexing experience of Mr Harris, who longed to leave the nursing home but chose to go back to it during his social leave? Mr Harris was able to clearly voice his resentment over the constraints of living in a secure care facility, and yet he also evidently found reassurance and comfort in its purposefully designed and structured environment and the assistance it offered him. I was confronted with questions: where was *home* for people like Mr Harris? Did Mr Harris feel more at home in the nursing home than in his daughter's house? What is the best way to care for Mr Harris and other residents like him who live out the final phase of their lives in nursing homes? This is a book about the complexity of living and ageing in a nursing home.[1] It is an enquiry that is of critical relevance to those who care for the aged, in professional or informal capacities as healthcare or aged care staff, or as relatives or friends of residents. The fieldwork I carried out considered the diverse ailments and different care structures I encountered with a particular group of people in a particular location; however, it speaks to a vast and growing audience. In ageing societies across the world, where a growing percentage of the population is experiencing physical and cognitive decline, the question of how best to care for the aged is one that increasingly affects us all.

I intend to show that it is possible for older people to live a good life in a nursing home if they can be assisted to do the things that they want to do with their bodies but are unable to do on their own. In conducting twelve months of fieldwork in two residential aged care facilities in metropolitan Adelaide, South Australia and then writing my understandings into this book, I came to realise how older people like Mr Harris could feel at home by being assisted to move. As this book will show, the location where older people receive care matters, but it does not determine whether they feel at home. Disease and decline affect people's experience of life as they age, and what may be characterized as 'the good life' in one's youth continually shifts and is always contingent on social and material circumstance. So what may largely be considered good for healthy and able-bodied people, such as spending a weekend away with family, may not be experienced as good for people with Parkinson's disease. Mr Harris could not manoeuvre his walker easily in his daughter's house, in rooms cluttered with furniture. Constricted in this way, he could not walk with this essential aid. Nor could he walk without it. With no handrails lining walls and corridors, he had nothing to hold on to. Off balance and unable to firmly put one foot in front of the other, he could not walk freely or feel safe in his daughter's house. He felt safer in the nursing home environment, where aid devices were available and staff readily came to his assistance. Rather than asking where home is located for older people like Mr Harris, this book follows the daily movements of some nursing home residents to understand how, with the right sort of assistance, they might come to experience a good quality of life. It traces the forms of care that can support them to feel 'all right' in a nursing home.

Movement capability is strongly related to admission into residential aged care. Mr Harris was admitted into the aged care facility due to the progression of his Parkinson's disease. After his wife died, he lived alone but after having frequent falls, tripping over rugs and his own feet, Mr Harris and his family felt that living independently at home was no longer an option for him. He was having difficulty with walking safely, needing someone to stand by his side to assist when he was struggling to balance. Because Mr Harris needed continual supervision and assistance to walk, a 'home care package'– tailored services designed to support elderly people to keep living in their own homes – was inadequate. Many nursing home residents will have been previously hospitalized due to injuries from falls before their admission into an aged care facility. This is a common pathway for the 1 in 20 elderly Australians who live in residential aged care facilities, according to the Australian Bureau of Statistics 2016 report on disability, ageing and carers (ABS 2016). In the current aged care system, home care packages and different levels of residential care provide senior Australians with options for nursing care and daily life assistance. Residential aged care is often seen as the last resort for care and support with daily living, yet it is usually turned to if assistance from family carers is not available.[2]

In aged care policy and research, a good life for older people is often conceptualized around the ideal of self-determination, which is all about autonomy – having control and choice over one's own life. However, moving into a nursing home is rarely perceived by the elderly as a decision that they willingly make on their own. Mr Harris entered the nursing home not out of choice but as a solution to his increasing inability to move around safely on his own. He hated the idea of living in a 'Home', but given his bodily condition, there was, he told me, no way to fight it. Although he entered residential care with his own consent, Mr Harris was forever resentful about being institutionalized. 'I want to go home,' he repeatedly complained. Residents often expressed their wish to go home, especially in the transition process of adjusting to life in the nursing home. Time and again they criticized the surveillance measures that restricted their movements in their new abode. Confronted with locked doors, security codes and the watchful eye of care staff and management, Mr Harris felt anything but 'at home'. In expressing his desire to go home, Mr Harris repeated his idea that the nursing home was a place in which he felt constrained – he did not feel 'right' there, and he wished he were free to leave. For Mr Harris and residents like him, home is less about bricks and mortar and more about a sense of being 'all right' in the living environment: being supported to move safely, to reach out to people and things in his surroundings, and to feel comfortable.

But despite wishing to leave the institution and to go home, Mr Harris could not feel at home in his daughter's house, where he felt even less comfortable – he later explained to me that he did not feel right there as he had 'no way to walk around'. At the core of Mr Harris feeling right and at home was his need and desire to walk freely as he wished. 'Going home', then, could be seen as a metaphor expressing his wish to find a way to feel all right – a sense of rightness of being. Though Mr Harris clearly voiced his resentment about having to live in a secure care facility, he also felt right there, especially on occasions when he was assisted to walk safely in that familiar environment.

As time passed during my research in the field, I noticed that all residents experienced an innermost drive to move, to connect and to stay in touch with the world. Yet, in studying the day-to-day lives of these residents, I also observed the loss of sensory capacities, motor coordination, balance and strength. Bodies increasingly became numb, weak, slow and unstable, and this limited their possibilities to act in the world in ways that they wished. I realized that the realities of physical and cognitive decline appear at odds with narratives of 'self-determination' that circulate in aged care policy and research. Movement for residents was not really about choice and control over one's own life. Rather, it was a matter of working interdependently with other people and things, simply to enable bodies to move. I saw that it was often through the most mundane everyday activities, like changing position from sitting to standing, walking or eating, that residents could, despite their bodily limitations, feel cared for and at home in the nursing home. These were occasions when Mrs Wilson could stand up on her own from an adjustable chair, Mrs Brie could eat from a lipped plate, and Mr Harris had his Parkinson's medication on time and, with the aid of care workers and his walker, could move freely around the facility.

For nursing home residents to feel a sense of being-at-home, they need the kind of care that responds to their innermost drive to move, by generating for them new ways of walking with relative ease. I call this kind of care 'right care'. The purpose of this book is thus to help those who care for older people to practise right care by understanding what right care is and how to deliver it in the context of residential aged care. I will do so by pointing to some important differences – different understandings of people' needs, and different experiences of care that older people receive in the nursing homes.

## Right Care

Care that is responsive to residents' bodies and needs is at the core of residents' experiences of feeling right in the nursing home. It happened when residents' need to move was attended to, such as when an arm reached out to support them to stand upright, or a walker was conveniently placed within reach, or a carer took time and used a gentle hand to get them dressed: all instances where vis-à-vis attentiveness and care from others allowed residents to continue doing the things that they wanted to do but were unable to do independently. On these occasions, when concerns had been taken care of, residents spoke of things 'working out all right' and of feeling 'just right', despite any difficulties to do with their bodies, communal living or institutional practices. Feeling just right and at ease, a sense of being in the right place, among the right objects, with the right persons, or being assisted at the right time in the right ways, was a constant theme of conversations at the nursing home; it is key to how residents feel, think and talk about being 'at home' in residential care.

Nevertheless, older people may not feel right while receiving care in the existing system. In September 2018, the Australian Broadcasting Corporation's (ABC) current events programme *Four Corners* aired a two-part documentary called 'Who Cares?' It presented a disturbing insight into the lives of those living in residential aged care facilities, highlighting examples of isolation and neglect. Following a number of reviews of aged care, and media exposure of poor care in the aged care system, the Royal Commission into Aged Care Quality and Safety was established to examine the quality of aged care services in Australia and whether those services are meeting the needs of the community.

Mr Anthony O'Donnell, who lives in residential aged care, gave evidence to the Royal Commission into Aged Care Quality and Safety. He said:

> The definition of care on both daytime shifts seems to be centred on making sure that there is something formally set down to do as a series of tasks. ... In one sense while immediate needs may well be met in this way, if considered objectively and without any intrusive thoughts about costs and the like, then such a definition of care is little more than is given to our sheep or cattle in the export business. (Pagone and Briggs 2021: 222)

Ms Johnson, another nursing home resident, also gave evidence to the Royal Commission, describing how staff members would enter her room as if she were not there, continuing their conversations with each other: 'Often not a word is said to me. I feel as though I am just an object that has to be moved from A to B' (Pagone and Briggs 2021: 222).

These narratives, drawn from the commission's Final Report, illustrate how care provided in the existing system can leave nursing home residents feeling dehumanized, isolated and ignored when they are handled and processed like a passive object, as staff tick off their tasks. During my fieldwork, residents talked about this task-based approach to care provision as staff 'doing care work'. Itemized as tasks to be completed, this form of 'care work' could actually contradict the essential meaning of care. In a task-orientated approach to care, staff strictly follow work schedules without being able to respond to residents in the moment – to their spontaneous efforts to move, to participate in the activities of daily living, to feel all right and at home. There can be a disjuncture between how care is conceived in aged care plans and procedures and fulfilling the actual needs of residents to be assisted to move with care. In other words, the kind of care that staff routinely carry out as tasks may not be the kind of care that residents need or want.

### *Introducing Assemblages*

This is a book about human and non-human actors and how they come together in different ways to enable different sorts of care, tailored to different bodies and levels of disability. Home, as this book will show, was made possible when the right elements came together at the right time to produce specific movements, senses and feelings. Home, as I will demonstrate, was a matter of moving and of being moved, with the right sorts of care, of shaping and of being shaped by one's body and one's world, and it is intimately connected to other people and things in what has been called an 'assemblage' (Deleuze and Guattari 1988).

It is important to describe the variety of things that can comprise these assemblages, many of which are centrally placed in the day-to-day lives of nursing home residents. Some tangible things, such as mobility aids and handrails installed in corridors, obviously play a pivotal role in supporting residents' efforts to move. A 4-wheeled walker is designed to provide balance to users when walking; it makes it easier for residents who have issues with stability to get around. Similarly, a modified armchair can provide optimum hip support and assist in standing and transfers when it is designed with adjustable seat height and angle and comfortable padded armrests. A special plate with built-up rims and ridges allows residents to more easily manage their food by fork or spoon. It works well for residents with low vision or for those who have difficulty grasping and manipulating eating utensils.

Technologies such as a call bell and sensor mat alarm systems are widely used in nursing homes to facilitate the connection between residents and staff. Such systems allow residents to alert staff when they need assistance. A call bell can be wired and installed in residents' rooms or be wireless and worn on the person. The call bell system displays the room number on staff deck phones, monitors in the nurses' station and LCD screens in corridors when a resident presses their button. A pressure-sensitive mat is a rubber mat with embedded electronic wires. It is used in nursing homes as a fall prevention strategy to monitor vulnerable residents' movements. Staff are required to give a quick response to sensor mat alarms by attending immediately to the resident.

Alongside this diverse range of technologies, nursing home residents spend most of their last years or months being attended to by personal care workers. Their job is physically demanding, and it calls for their own bodies to move in response to residents' movements. Whether walking or eating, putting feet on the carpet or food in the mouth, the interlaced hands of care staff and residents come together as one, co-functioning in an assemblage. In examining how these people and things come together, this book shows how a sense of home comes from residents' everyday movements, which are intimately entwined in the relational social world of the nursing home.

The assistive devices, medications and staff assistance that support residents to move are all part of the provision of care services in nursing homes and are routinely delivered within the limits of care plans and aged care funding policy. However, while staff, medications and aid equipment can be assembled to support residents to move, they can also restrain residents from moving. For example, residents are often seated in 'princess chairs', pressure-cushioned chairs that are designed with a curved backrest to provide extra postural support and comfort for residents sitting for long hours. On the other hand, being left sitting in this chair for long periods can restrain voluntary movement or prevent the person from engaging with other residents.

The term 'care' is understood in this study as being made up of not one but multiple assemblages of care. Using the Deleuzian concept of assemblage, I analyse how elderly residents' movements meshed with multiple entities, including staff, medications, walking aids, assistive utensils, adjustable beds and chairs, as well as aged care policies, assessments, care plans and fall prevention programmes. I will show how some components are assembled productively, to facilitate the movements residents wish to make, and conversely, how other assemblages could be counterproductive, such as certain discourses of risk or agitation, which could be used to restrain people and inhibit movement. I outline what I believe are productive and right 'assemblages of care' (Musolino 2016) and explore the tension between how care is presently conceived – in the contexts of policies and care plans – and how, conversely, it could be practised; for example, by assisting residents to make movements they feel they cannot make on their own, in ways that would feel right to them.

## *Care That 'Works All Right'*

This book attempts to describe and understand care not as 'care work' but as what works so that residents may actually feel cared for, at ease and at home. Bodily impairments create blockages that lead to ruptures in movement: incomplete attempts to stand or to walk by smoothly putting one foot in front of the other. Enabling movement was, for residents and staff, a matter of assembling the right people and things so that 'bad knees', 'weak legs' or 'diabetic feet' can, as staff said, 'work all right'. The word 'right' was frequently used by staff to refer to situations when residents were observed to be able to move with just the right type and amount of assistance. These were occasions when a walker became 'just right', or the assemblage of a staff-assisted walking routine and medication schedule were delivered on time. As I will detail in Chapter 1 of this book, using the example of Mrs Casey, care that 'works all right' depends on synthesized efforts. In this case, extra funding was invested by the service provider to hire a physiotherapist and assistant. Mrs Casey's wish to relearn to walk was supported by the integrated care management team in the form of allocated staff time; and her efforts to walk joined with those of allied health professionals and personal care staff.

In the nursing homes, I could see how care that enabled residents to feel right was not delivered *because of* the system but *in spite of* the system. It was delivered if and when situations were favourable and staff were free to respond to individual residents' needs. Right care is what works, and what works for residents requires shifting arrangements of people and things coming together to 'step in' or 'lend a hand', often outside of their time-poor work schedules. Right assemblages of care cannot be fixed or documented easily in care plans. Adjustments need to be made constantly, depending on the vicissitudes of bodies and situations. Right assemblages of care require constant 'tinkering' from one moment to the next' (Mol, Moser and Pols 2010).

While Mol et al. (2010) have examined tinkering practices and technologies as a way into theorizing the nature of care, the theme of power, developed by Martin and colleagues (2015: 628), is also useful for analysing how caregiving involves a complex entanglement of multiple things and people, amid asymmetrical power relations. Thinking about power as entailed in affective dis/engagements through multisensory modes and means enables sensory analysis (Dennis 2018) of how power relates to care, and is thus always entailed in the question of how residents become at home in nursing homes.

## *Caring beyond the Limits*

Within biomedical framings of ageing, the aged are regarded by health professionals as people struggling with physical limitations: declining bodies, damaged bodies, bodies that are painful, insensible, slowed down or in stasis. As the process of deterioration is irreversible, ageing bodies will inevitably fail to function at some stage. The widespread equation of old age with disease has led to the medicalization of old age and death, from which perspective the aged are viewed as frail, often mentally impaired and otherwise limited in human capabilities. As Kaufman points out: 'Old age-as-disease has become a more compelling "truth" than old age as one of several normal developmental processes' (1994a: 432). Defined as 'older adults or aged individuals who are lacking in general strength and who are unusually susceptible to disease or to other infirmity' (Bergman et al. 2007: 731–32), the term 'frail elderly' has become a medical concept associated with disease and disability. Culturally conceived as regression, old age is made equivalent to decline. Nonetheless, as revealed in Kaufman's discussion of frailty beyond instrumental definitions, frailty is a lived problem that is socially constructed as a parameter of risk for institutionalization (1994b: 54–56).

Difficulties with daily life activities and normal functioning are understood in physiological research as the result of the ageing process, characterized by reduced functional capacities. This is most obvious in how residents' difficulties with walking are biomedically constructed into a loss of bodily sensitivity, flexibility, strength and coordination. In this singular attention to biological aspects of ageing, decreased function is foregrounded and is presented as natural and inevitable. Yet, this direct association of bodily decline with loss of capacity in old age is at odds with the complexities of movements that I observed in the day-to-day lives of nursing home residents. What is missing in this approach is how elderly people can actively adapt and adjust to bodily changes in their real-world environments, and how the right care can enable people to develop new ways of moving with relative ease.

The mental deficit associated with age has been among the most deeply stigmatized conditions in human history (Cohen 2006). It is also viewed as a medical issue first and foremost (Ballenger 2006: 106). Since German physician Alois Alzheimer first discovered the dramatic shrinkage and abnormal structures in the brain of his patient Auguste D. in 1906, a condition that was coined as Alzheimer's disease by psychiatrist Emil Kraepelin in 1910, dementia has largely been studied and defined through biomedical discourse. In biomedicine, dementia is conceptualized as a highly disabling neurological condition that is, according to the Australian Institute of Health and Welfare, not curable by medical intervention (AIHW 2007). In her compelling book, *The Alzheimer Conundrum*, Margaret Lock (2013) gives a provocative account of why Alzheimer's disease is such a puzzling mix of scientific hypotheses, research agendas, pharmaceutical interests, funding objectives and theories of ageing. She highlights just how much we do not know, from problems with Alzheimer's pathology, testing and diagnosis, to the search for drug treatment. Nonetheless, with its genetic, diagnostic and predictive uncertainties, the usual biomedical discourse about Alzheimer's disease shapes how people perceive and understand the experiences of those who are affected. In relation to dementia diagnosis, people use such references as the 'gothic and zombie stories' or the 'horror of Alzheimer's' (Taylor 2008: 317, 324). People with dementia are regarded as suffering a loss of both mind and self – as people incapable of rational communication or maintaining relationships. What Cohen (1998) terms as 'senility' has been 'reduced' to a medical problem, a progressive and terminal cognitive disease, within the rigid logic of dementia diagnosis and care (Cohen 2006: 3).

The biomedical construction of dementia diagnosis is to focus on brain pathology and symptoms of cognitive decline, which focus on impairments. These include: lack of capability in logical reasoning, planning, and ability to focus on intentional and purposive activity; decreased ability to be attentional, reflective, to form short-term memories or access long-term memories, such as autobiographical memory, as well as to communicate effectively using language. If we construct dementia as a cognitive disease, its biomedical framing poses a threat to the traditional concept of personhood, which is centred around cognition. In this model, one relates to other things and beings as a 'self' through a mind where meanings – symbolic representations of objects, events and relations – are generated in linguistic forms for reflection and communication. A functioning mind is considered central to a meaningful existence of being able to sustain relationships with others in the world. Thinking about dementia in terms of brain pathology and symptoms of cognitive decline, dementia is seen in terms of loss: of mind, of self and of a meaningful existence in relation to other people and things.

In nursing homes, residents in the later stages of dementia are often described by some staff as 'dementia full stop', a phrase that suggests futility and finality. In this version of dementia, personhood is disintegrated and eventually dissolves into disease itself. Drawing on Erving Goffman's (1961) conception of mortification, Neil Henderson argues in his ethnographic work on a dementia unit that the institutional 'induction process designed to kill the prior social self and remake the person into another entity congenial to the goals of the new environment' marks the social death of the person (2003: 154). This represents the first burial (Kayser-Jones 2003: 66; Stafford 2003a: 17) before the person's second, biological death.

The power of biomedical framing 'reaches into the very grain of individuals, touches their bodies and inserts itself into their actions and attitudes, their discourses, learning processes and everyday lives' (Foucault 1980: 39). When care is disease-centred, the lived experiences of people with dementia are perceived and understood as symptoms. Focusing on mental loss, their speech and movements are classed as 'behaviours' that are void of meaning. When their behaviours are thought to be excessive, persistent or harmful to other people and themselves, those behaviours are further constructed as 'behavioural problems', the behavioural and psychological symptoms of dementia, which require drug treatment or psychosocial intervention. As long as the lived experiences of people with dementia are biomedically constructed into symptoms that are pathological and abnormal, these constructs will affect how these people are cared for. This book will show how discourses of 'mindless' bodies or 'meaningless' movement promote the restrictive practices of fall prevention that often translate into restraint on aged care residents.

Biomedical framings and contemporary social imaginings of ageing and age-related decline limit our understanding of what can be made possible for elderly people to live a good life despite their various conditions and situations. While the notion of care is represented in aged care policy as a way of enhancing people's physical and cognitive capacities by extending the limits of what is possible for people who are severely impaired or dying, in practice care is often reduced to strict biomedical constructs. In contrast, this book advocates a rethink on what is 'reasonably possible' for the elderly by looking beyond biomedical understandings. My fieldwork with residents with a range of physical and mental disabilities (due to various forms and stages of dementia) enabled me to record and analyse the variety of their experiences, as well as to critically reflect on the surrounding ethics, politics and operationalization of care in the nursing homes.

In his conceptualization of a social ethics of care, Rapport (2018) draws on Jackson's (1995) notion of 'home' to emphasize how caring for the elderly is imperative to their achieving a sense of being-at-home-in-the-world. He points to the tension between 'being for oneself and being for others' and suggests that even as they are being cared for the elderly may simultaneously be constrained from exercising their free will. He thus argues that care needs to be a matter of upholding the 'personal preserve' of the elderly and 'caring that their autonomy is not infringed: that [is] so far as possible, and for as long as possible' (Rapport 2018: 255–56). Rapport's argument that care needs to be a matter of protecting the elderly's autonomy is critical to thinking about care for people with dementia. Yet, within

Rapport's conceptual framework of social ethics of care, it is difficult to situate an ethical form of care for residents with cognitive impairments due to late-stage dementia. With its emphasis on cognitive capacity, his conception of 'personal preserve' is really only applicable to people who have mental competence.

In this ethnography on the minutiae of nursing home residents' movements, I argue that autonomy needs to be understood as something more than conscious choice and action. I examine the potential benefits of resident-staff-assistive technology assemblages to provide new knowledge about how people with dementia can still relate to others, not cognitively but sensorially and affectively, through movement.

## Theoretical Directions: Becoming-at-Home in Movement

Writing from different theoretical perspectives, ageing and care-related studies frequently draw on the concept of home to think about older people's lives. The etymology of the word 'home' in both German and English shows a close association between house, or a dwelling place, and home in the material sense. Contemporary Eurocentric conceptions of home suggest a physical structure or dwelling. Founded on the distinction between public and private, and the inside and outside world, home is also conceived as a haven, a confined space that offers freedom and control, security, an intimate context for close, caring relationships and scope for creativity and regeneration. Related to this concept of home is the idea that it is an enclosed, private and domestic space, clearly differentiated from public space and shielded from public scrutiny and surveillance (Mallett 2004).

Unlike the notion of home as a domestic space, the nursing home is conceived as a contested cultural space 'composed of elements drawn from oppositional spheres of meaning: home and hospital' (Stafford 2003b: 121). It conflates the practice of nursing and the place of home. The combination of a medical institution with a residential facility is thought to have created a categorical ambiguity for people living and working there. While the concept of 'home' has the connotations of private property, independent living, domestic setting and intimate relationships, the concept of 'nursing' is associated with the fragility, disability and decline of aged bodies, and the 'bed-and-body work' involved in an institutional care setting (Diamond 1992; Gubrium 1975: 123). This contradictory meaning is seen by Stafford as 'the chief problematic of the nursing home – its *inherent cultural ambiguity*' (2003a: 8; italics original). Extending Stafford's illustration of the nursing home as possessing the dual character of home (in that older persons are residents) and hospital (in that older persons are patients),

Bland (2007: 941) claims that nursing homes have two additional characteristics: that of hotel (in that older persons are customers) and as hospice, a place for those who are dying. Seen in this way, the institution is a hybrid of all four characterizations.

Researchers often frame their nursing home studies, explicitly or implicitly, within the relationship between home and nursing home and tend to focus on the movement of people from the home to the nursing home; that is, about making a transition from one place to another. Some researchers consider moving into residential care as a rupture, 'a transition from "doing for" to "being done for", as well as a transition from independence to dependence' (Higgins 1989: 141). In the analysis of the transition as a rupture and displacement from home, home and nursing home are conceived as two opposing concepts, domains or sociocultural spaces. The focus is often around the structures and practices at the institutional level (such as the care culture, routine practice and built design), which are seen as having significant influence on residents' lives. The transition from home to the nursing home is widely seen to involve multiple forms of loss – displacement from the family home, dispossession of pre-loved objects and dissociation from loved ones – leading to an overwhelming sense of withdrawal and disconnection. The loss incurred in the transition to nursing home life is often thought of as irreversible because residents can neither re-create their home in a nursing home or return to their own homes. The majority will eventually die in nursing homes, and with escalating dependence on assistance, tools and facilities, residents are portrayed as being a burden, increasingly helpless and lacking in autonomy.

The notion of home and nursing home as fixed and finished structural entities is increasingly questioned in contemporary research. Some researchers position home and the nursing home not in opposition but as relational concepts held in tension. They highlight potential continuities of life before and after the move into the nursing home by incorporating what was in the residents' prior existence, including personal histories, possessions, family and social relations, into their existential present. With a shift of focus from rupture to continuity, researchers gradually come to understand home as a *sense of home* and describe how home is felt and thought.

For theorists on home, a sense of home is made not only through social and discursive constructs as meanings but also through lived experience as senses and feelings (Ahmed 1999; Gurney 1997; M. Jackson 1995; Somerville 1992). As life goes on, a different sense of home may evolve over time. It can be oriented to production, a sense of security, stability and belonging; it can also be experienced as a sense of defence, protection and autonomy, as conveyed in the nineteenth-century saying, 'The Englishman's house is his castle'. The domestic environment is thought to imbue elderly people with a sense of control; it is where they can interact with their own long-held possessions and thus retain important memories.

Nursing homes today have evolved into a more home-like environments through their architectural and interior design. Residential aged care facilities encourage residents to bring personal possessions with them as an initiative intended to create a sense of continuity of life before and after nursing home placement. In both facilities where I did my fieldwork, I noted that on admission residents were encouraged to personalize their rooms using their own furniture, souvenirs and photos of families and pets (see Illustration 0.1). It is assumed that these objects from their former homes can help to transfer a sense of personal identity, home and belonging to their new lives in an unfamiliar institutional setting (Cram and Paton 1993; Rowles 1993). In discussions about what it means to retain a sense of home, researchers often refer to the objects, beings or relationships (such as with their beloved pets; see Illustration 0.2) that came from home and moved with people into the nursing homes.

Arguing that objects are not just passive symbols representing a sense of home, Lovatt wrote that it is not the objects themselves but the interactions between residents and these objects that enable residents to feel at home while 'doing home' (2018: 366). By the term 'doing home', Lovatt refers to a particular set of regular practices and routines, including acquiring new things, displaying existing possessions, and everyday domestic practices such as cleaning and hosting guests.

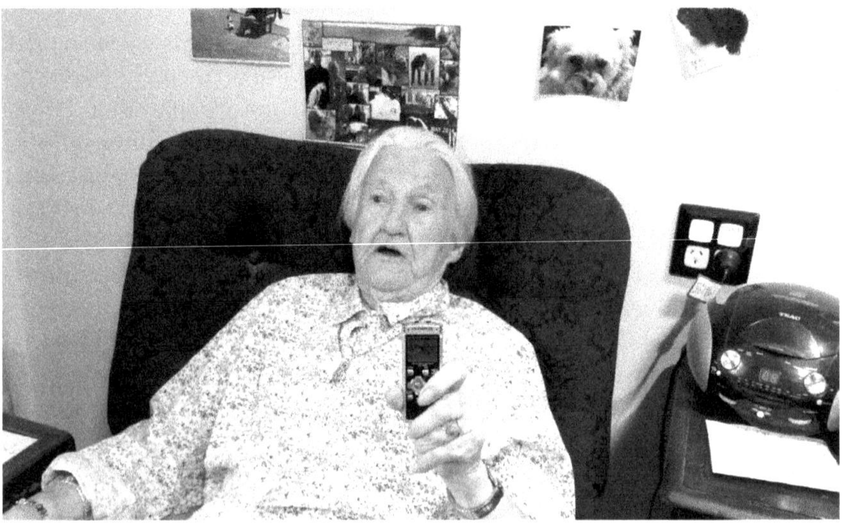

**ILLUSTRATION 0.1.** A resident interviewed in her room in the aged care facility in 2015. © Angela Zhang.

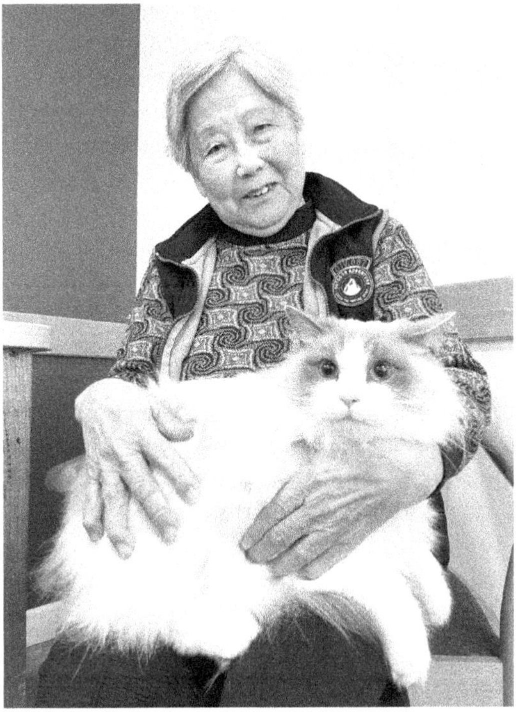

**ILLUSTRATION 0.2.** A resident and her cat in the aged care facility. Image provided courtesy of Elder Chinese Home.

With a shift of focus away from the physical surroundings where elderly people live and the objects that they possess, researchers are increasingly placing their study focus on individual residents and their own efforts to adapt to nursing home environments. Nursing home residents are often portrayed as being able to settle into their lives in nursing homes with a sense of peace, stabilization and satisfaction. As Minney and Ranzijn reported in their study on a South Australian nursing home, one resident grieved the loss of her beautiful home, but said, 'I think I'm happier here' (2015: 919). With a life that is as close as possible to that lived before admission, elderly people, according to these studies, 'regain normality', maintaining their individual 'sense of biography, of self and of belonging' (Nolan et al. 1996: 271).

In describing practices of 'doing home' as residents transition to their new lives in residential care, researchers look for threads of continuity in what residents themselves do in order to adjust. This approach views the transition from home to nursing home as the process of becoming-at-home. Drawing on Allan and Crow's theory of 'becoming at home' as 'essentially an active process which involves "housework" in the broadest sense of that term' (1989: 11). Lovatt suggests that a feeling of belonging and a sense of control comes from the effort that residents make to incorporate objects from a previous life into their new nursing home environment. It is further argued that being-at-home in a nursing home need not be so different from being-at-home at other stages of the life course and in other settings (2018: 375). For this to be true, the way that people feel and experience home would have to remain largely the same across different stages and settings of life.

However, residents' ability to manage everyday activities is affected over the course of their lives by their bodily conditions. Bodily deterioration accelerates in the latter stages of life. In failing to consider how ageing affects us physically as we go through life's stages, an important dimension of change is ignored. Although some research suggests that physical disabilities do not necessarily prevent residents from living active lives, the impact of bodily deterioration is captured in other studies and has been conveyed using residents' own narratives. Lily Robinson, a nursing home resident interviewed by Gubrium, contrasted her experience as a 'whole being' at home with her sense of 'being partial' living in a nursing home, regretting her inability to 'take care of everything' after the amputation of her legs (1993: 128–29).

The effort required to carry out daily activities is also affected by residents' material surroundings. Whether or not material things (e.g. an electric kettle or a toaster) can be made available to a resident (with or without signs of cognitive impairments) and how these material things should be provided (temporarily or permanently) and used (supervised or unsupervised) vary in different settings and permutations. Similar to the multidimensional home, as a site of caregiving, a nursing home is also a multidimensional institution, a site of contestation and complexity, made up of residents' regular practices, routines and interactions with their material surroundings. While in Lovatt's study residents could exercise a level of choice over which material things were provided in their individual rooms, acquisition of these material things was only made possible with the support of facility management and staff. Similarly, how various forms of assistance are provided (or not) impacts on residents' re-creation of a sense of home in the nursing home. Individual efforts to re-create home are always made according to the availability of supportive material things and persons, such as aid devices and carers.

This book has at its heart the lived experience of residents' declining bodies, specifically the care they need to enable them to move. As we know, and this book will show, ageing affects bodies; thus living out the final stages of one's life in a nursing home is not the same as living at earlier stages of one's life course. And yet residents in this study could often re-create a sense of home through the most mundane everyday activity – that of venturing to walk beyond the physical confines of their rooms. Instead of interacting just with objects within their rooms, residents moved beyond their personal quarters. With the help of assistive hands and mobility aids, they could be physically in touch with objects in communal areas: handrails in the corridors, or tables and chairs in the lounge and dining areas. Conceptualizing home in terms of household objects, which must, by definition, relate to domestic objects in residents' rooms, can be simplistic and reductive, as that definition cannot accommodate the complex and productive interrelationships between residents and other people and fittings in the wider nursing home environment, such as carpeted floors, grab-rails and corridors. As will be shown, the feeling of being-at-home emerges through the lived experience of being in contact with other people and other objects in the nursing home. When other bodies and material things support and respond to residents' attempts to move, this can lead to an overall feeling of satisfaction and wellbeing. It is precisely at this point that this study takes a departure from the existing literature on *what* home means to individual residents, to foreground instead the relational and embodied experience of *how* home is experienced in residential care. Although residents with severe physical or cognitive impairments could no longer carry out the routine activities that may conform to the usual idea of 'doing home', they could still experience a sense of home in the nursing home. This book explores what this means by investigating to what extent residents with different bodily conditions, including those with and without cognitive impairments, and with different medical conditions and disease trajectories, are able to move.

A sense of home will not be examined here through the lens of transition, which treats the idea of moving from home to residential care as an inevitable rupture, nor will it be explained in terms of objects or practices that inspire memories of a previous home. Instead, I shift my focus towards the *everyday movements* that residents in care are able to make. I hold the view that life continues across home and the nursing home not because of particular possessions, persons or practices but because, even in care, people continue to live their everyday lives through walking, standing and eating – the ordinary daily movements that are fundamental to our being-in-the-world (Barbaras 2008; Ingold 2011).

For Merleau-Ponty, a living body is not only 'the ground of perceptual processes that end in objectification' but also a 'general power of inhabiting all the environments which the world contains' (Merleau-Ponty 1962: 311). Physical things and spaces can be incorporated into self on the motile, sensual, perceptual level by means of sensory extension through multisensory processes (Dennis 2007). For Dennis (2004), sensory extension or contraction gives rise to feelings of joy or pain. Approaching movement through the notion of sensory extension leads to the understanding of movement as both sensorial and affective. Dennis's notion of sensory extension is a form of relational extension (Latimer and Munro 2009): establishing person–world connectedness through routine practices in order to create a sense of belonging.

For Barbaras, life as such 'must be understood as movement in a radicalized sense, in which the living being is no more the subject than the product' (Barbaras 2008: 3). To understand life as the original unity of the living being and the lived experience across the conscious and preconscious levels, Barbaras proposes a third mode in which being is movement (2008: 8). He suggests that movement is the manifestation of the life of a living being, 'a moment of accomplishment [which] passes into exteriority because it is only realized through concrete movements' (Barbaras 2008: 14).

Ingold (2011, 2017) considers that being alive is a mode of moving through the world with others. He coins the term 'correspondence' (Ingold 2017: 9) to describe the dynamic processes of engaging with other material things and beings as attending to and responding to in and through movements. In the context of this book, correspondence can be seen as the process in and through which residents' efforts to move are joined by other supportive material things and persons. Ingold's notion of correspondence describes the processual formation of connectedness, through the exchanges of linguistic expressions between persons, or engagements between persons and things in co-movements, such as in walking together. Thinking about home in residential care through the theoretical concepts of perception (Merleau-Ponty 1962), sensory extension (Dennis 2004, 2007), movement (Barbaras 2008) and correspondence (Ingold 2017) confirms the importance of supporting a variety of experiences for residents in different states of bodily and/or cognitive decline.

Returning to the notion of home, the sense of rightness experienced by nursing home residents resonates with what Michael Jackson, an anthropologist who studied among Warlpiri people in central Australia, describes as 'a sense of existential control and connectedness' (1995: 154). For Jackson, home is not associated with any particular property, place, possession, person or practice. In his work *At Home in the World*, Jackson uses the term 'home' to describe people's experience of a reciprocal person–world relationship, whereby one retains some control over and connectedness with the world. Feeling 'at home in the world' emerges 'when what we do has some effect and what we say carries some weight' (1995: 123). Being-at-home is thus approached as a metaphor for the experience of trying to strike a balance between acting and being acted upon, and it is considered within a relational framework that can represent how people can assert themselves, to varying degrees, in the world. Of critical importance to Jackson's notion of home is the positioning of the need for a sense of connectedness and control as fundamental to human life. 'Home', in Jackson's sense of the term, is thus an 'existential imperative' (2002: 14).

My fieldwork results suggest that some residents experienced a sense of being-at-home in the nursing home. However, unlike Jackson's informants, participants in this study were hampered by ageing and dying bodies. They experienced the existential imperative, not as a need for some degree of choice or control over their own lives but primarily as an innermost drive to move. This study follows their footsteps and traces their attempts to move and to act in the world despite their various states of bodily and cognitive decline. Accordingly, I extend Jackson's (1995, 2002) notions of home and the existential imperative to the everyday experiences of nursing home residents with physical and/or cognitive impairments.

Moving beyond Jackson's assumption that persons share similar experiences of being physically or cognitively intact, I turn to Deleuze and Guattari's (1977, 1988) theories of becoming and desiring-production. Rather than understanding the world to be composed of relatively stable entities of things and beings, let us assume everything is in a state of motion, a process of becoming, a multiplicity (Deleuze and Guattari 1988). Becoming is thus not about what is already constituted and settled – subject or object, body or mind, wish or will – but about the shifting generative potentials made possible through desiring-production. In this sense, for aged and frail nursing home residents, walking is always a becoming-walking in which tensions between walking and not walking must be continuously negotiated. Drawing on Mol, Moser and Pols's (2010) work of care as a practice of tinkering, Puig de la Bellacasa (2011) and Martin, Myers and Viseu's (2015) work examining care through themes of power, and Rapport's (2018) notion of care as a balance between inclusion and autonomy, I want to show how right care, if it is to properly assist residents to have a sense of home, must be enacted differently, as multiplicities.

In this book, I set out to destabilize deficit models of ageing. The theory of desiring-production offers a useful analytic lens with which to examine how residents' stiff and sore bodies were set in motion in the actions of walking, standing and eating. The term 'desiring machine' (Deleuze and Guattari 1977) is used to describe how bodies and things come together in the process of desiring-production. A mouth is coupled with an edible thing, a pair of feet is paired with a surface to walk on; these become 'desiring machines', simultaneously affecting and affected, in connective and associative syntheses that induce movements and feelings. In walking or eating, the feet and the carpet, and the mouth, edibles and cutlery, respectively, come together as one, co-functioning in an assemblage

(Deleuze and Guattari 1988). The concept of assemblage is intimately related to 'becomings', processes in which disparate objects, beings, events and discourses co-exist as multiplicities through metamorphosis. Deleuze and Guattari's terms of productive desire, assemblage and multiplicity are useful linguistic hangers for thinking about and articulating how residents may be supported to become mobile and feel more at home. In sum, I propose here that home is a process of becoming-at-home-in-the-world, and I explore how becoming-at-home occurs through shifting and entangled movements made possible through assemblages of things and persons.

## The Nursing Homes

Fieldwork for this project occurred in two residential aged care facilities, Auxilia and Dulce Domum, situated in the suburbs of Adelaide, South Australia. Situated in an affluent area of Adelaide, Auxilia is a not-for-profit facility with over 150 government-subsidized aged care beds, while Dulce Domum, with around 80 beds, is affiliated to a large multistate aged care service provider in the private sector. The 230 residents living in these two care facilities had access to a wide range of amenities, including a community centre, café (see Illustration 0.3) and outdoor café (see Illustration 0.4), library, hairdressing salon (see Illustration 0.5), chapel (see Illustration 0.6), internet café and garden area (see Illustration 0.7).

Features such as the grand lobby, elevated interior decor, 'deluxe' rooms and polite well-trained staff were similar to those found in hotels. In that way, the commoditization of care is evident today in the aged care industry in Australia. Nevertheless, elderly Australians admitted into aged care facilities situated in less affluent suburbs may (and often do) live in environments that are quite different from those that form the background of this study. The 'standard' living condition in a nursing home can be quite basic, with resident bedrooms furnished with a single bed, a wardrobe, a locker and a chair, and residents may have to share a toilet and bathroom. Residents living in other facilities may not have access to the many on-site amenities that are referred to this study. I try to describe the nursing homes in this book accurately, but it is important to remember they are by no means representative of all aged care homes in Australia.

Consistent with the aged demographic in the two suburbs in which this research was undertaken, residents were mostly Anglo-European, had middle-class backgrounds, had been married, and there was a higher ratio of women to men. Most of the residents spoke English, even though some of them had difficulty with finding words or composing meaningful sentences due to cognitive impairments. Some overseas-born residents had

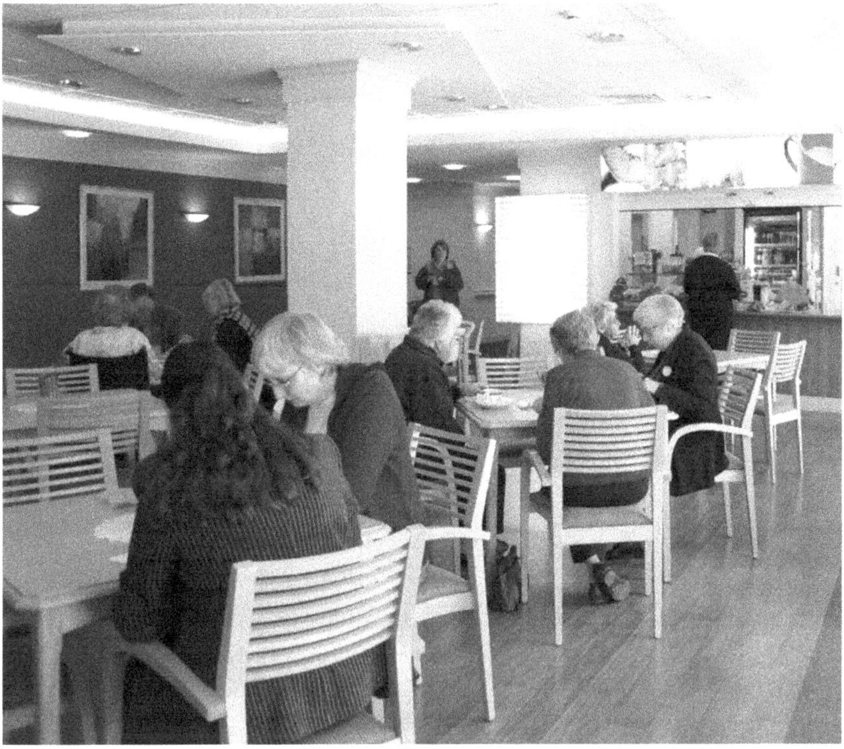

ILLUSTRATION 0.3. Residents receiving visiting family and friends in the on-site café. Image provided courtesy of Helpinghand.

lost their English proficiency and switched back to their mother tongue (e.g. German).

Staff composition in the two facilities was quite different in terms of gender, age and ethnicity. In Dulce Domum, staff were mostly young or middle-aged female migrant workers, while in Auxilia the staff cohort was older (a small proportion was close to retirement age, and several were still working casually after retirement) and more gender-balanced. There were significantly more middle-aged, both male and female, workers from the local communities employed in Auxilia.

## Moving, Observing and Describing in the Nursing Home

In this fieldwork-based study, I aimed to acquire a deep understanding of whether and how elderly Australians could feel at home in a nursing home during the last stages of life. I did so by attempting to feel in my own

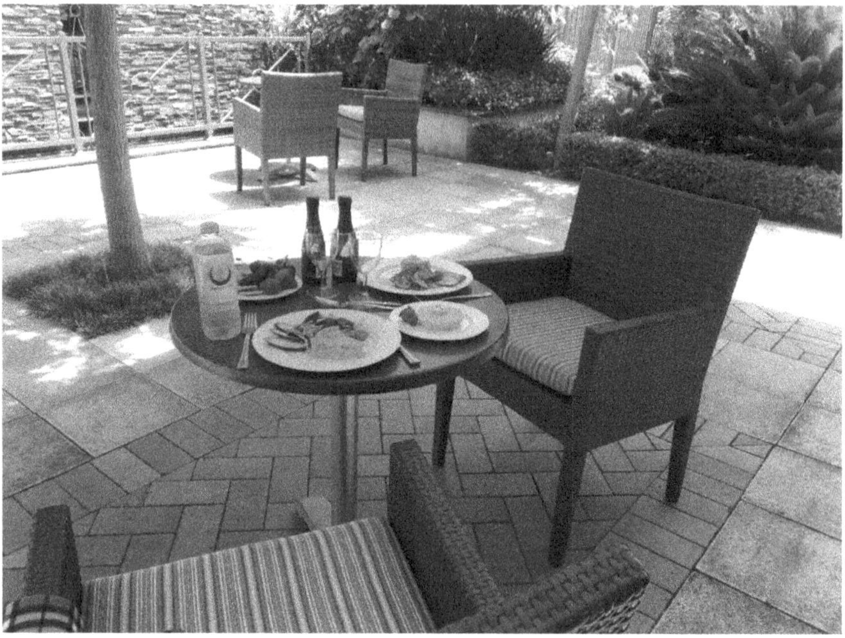

ILLUSTRATION 0.4. Outdoor café seating. Image provided courtesy of Helpinghand.

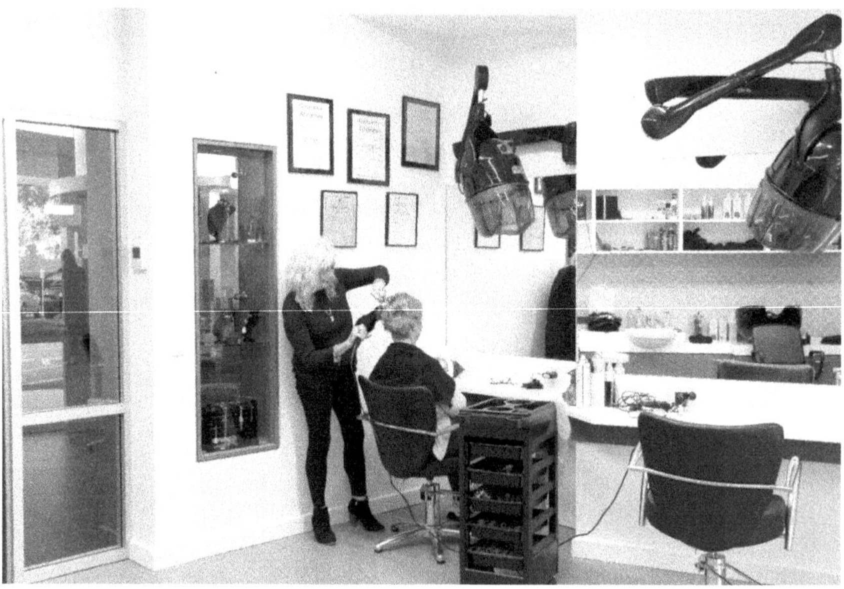

ILLUSTRATION 0.5. A hairdresser serving a resident in the on-site hair salon. Image provided courtesy of Helpinghand.

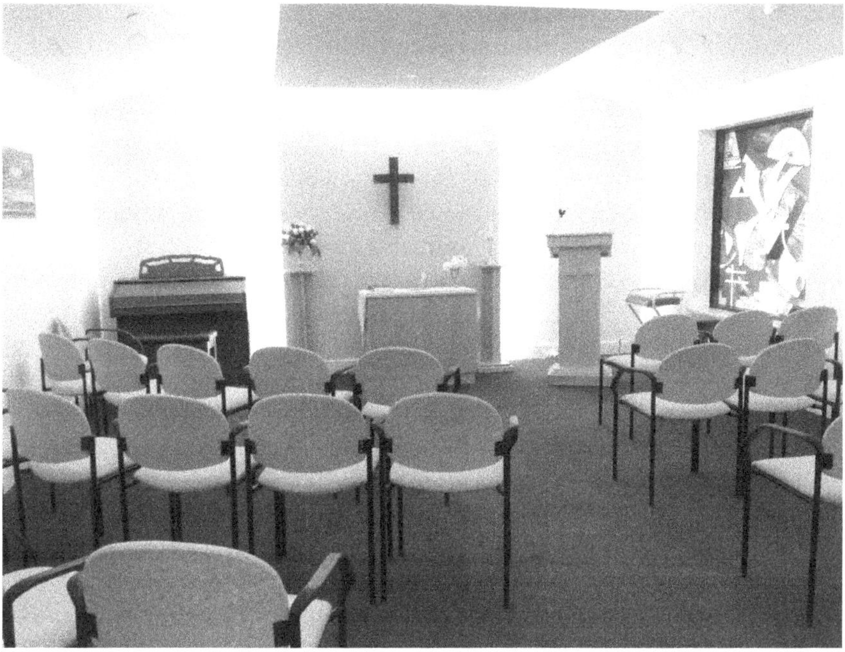

ILLUSTRATION 0.6. On-site chapel. Image provided courtesy of Helpinghand.

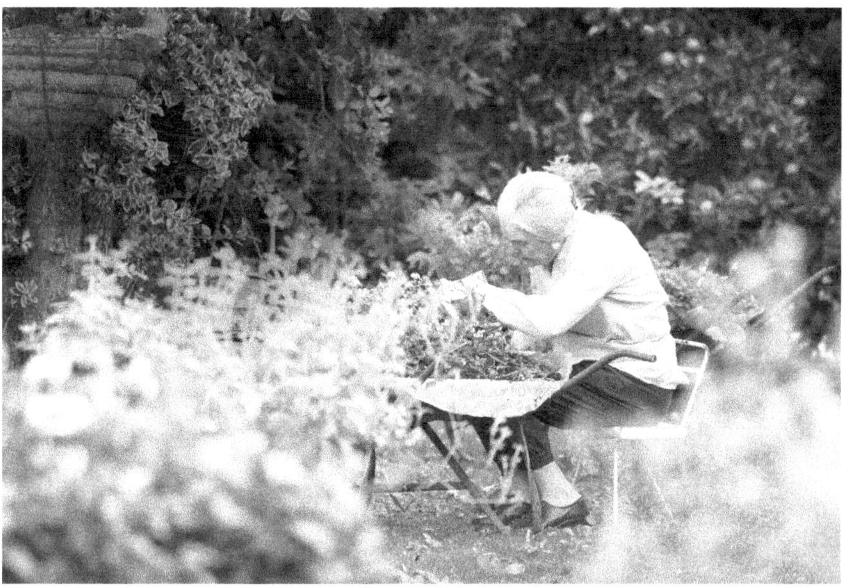

ILLUSTRATION 0.7. A resident gardening. Image provided courtesy of Helpinghand.

body the movements that residents and staff made so that I could share in them. The word 'understanding' here thus refers to the ethnographic insights I gained through experiencing other ways of moving and feeling and then reflecting on my experience. It would not, of course, enable me to intimately know the experience as if I were an aged care resident actually living that life. Rather, instead of exploring what it is like to be a nursing home resident, I set out to acquire a deep understanding of residents' ways of inhabiting nursing home environments.

Undergoing an immersive process of gradual familiarization and differentiation was key to my decision to use movement as the prime methodological vehicle. In this process of immersive participating, observing, reflecting, describing and communicating, staff-assisted residents' movements were felt, seen, thought through and discussed. The entire process was a scenario for me to have different experiences (being assisted by different staff members in different contexts), see things from different perspectives (of residents, physiotherapists, nurses and personal care workers) and assimilate different care practices (assessment, care planning and staff-assisted walking and transfers) into my developing understanding of how residents are assisted to move in the nursing homes.

This multifaceted, open-ended process involved multisensory engagement with various objects and persons, such as aiding devices, other equipment and staff, and the complex interplay of discourses (e.g. funding schemes, work efficiency, staff workload and resident risk and safety). As shown in the photograph taken during my fieldwork (see Illustration 0.8), at one stage I relearned how to walk with assistance from a physiotherapist and a walking frame. I videorecorded myself walking with assistance, and also walking to assist residents, so that I could later visualize the movements and processes.

In watching movements in context, I could relate how I felt while moving with what I observed while watching, to later reflect on the process and make it explicit through description and analysis. In playing multiple roles – walking like residents, walking with residents, observing residents and staff walking, and then writing a care plan for staff-assisted walking and transfer – I became attuned to a mix of sensory, affective and cognitive experience and could then draw ethnographic insights. In moving, touching, watching, and being moved, touched and watched, as Latour argues, the body may be thought of as 'an interface that becomes more and more describable as it learns to be affected by more and more elements' (2004: 206).

My bodily engagement in daily care delivery revealed to me the asymmetrical power relations entailed in the social institution of the nursing home. This was made apparent when I was assisted by two personal care

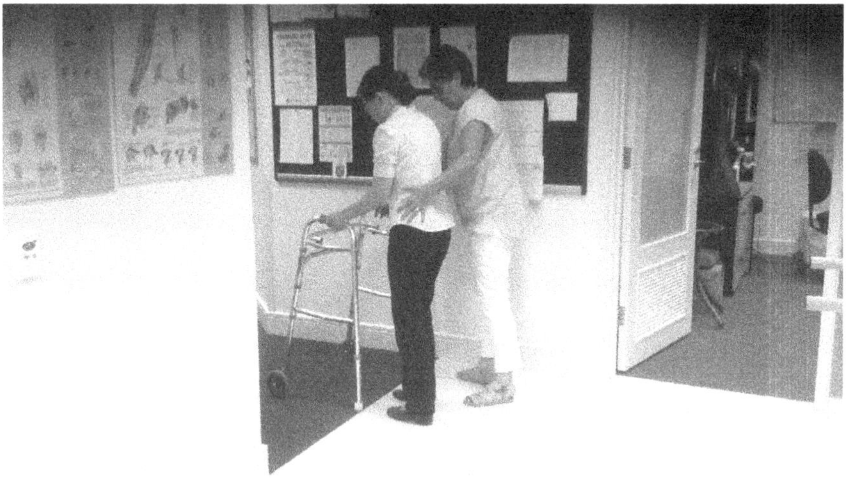

**ILLUSTRATION 0.8.** The ethnographer learning to walk with a walking frame and assistance from a physiotherapist in 2015. © Angela Zhang.

workers with transferring from bed to chair (See Illustration 0.8), an activity that requires both the resident and staff to exert some force in order to push, pull, lift and turn in coordinated movements. With two care workers standing on opposite sides of the bed and looking down at me from above, I instantly felt the dead weight of my body, given my supine position, and I experienced for the first time the vulnerability of being a care recipient. 'You are in our hands now', the carer (with whom I had made an acquaintance) said jokingly, as she held up her hands. This feeling of being weak and vulnerable was deepened later when I watched the videorecording, which showed the specific deployment of my body in relation to the bodies of the carers in vivid detail.

By being involved in the particular bodily relations applied by a particular social institution, as Lyon and Barbalet (1994) argue, one's own body can be extended into a certain social order through sensory modes and means. What characterizes bodily relations in the nursing home are the authorized and authoritative touches and gazes of staff upon a resident's body and the effects on the recipient of such intimate contact. In this situation, power infiltrates care. This was revealed to me when I was myself 'manually handled' at different times, and staff made various comments about my performance. When I was more responsive to staff movements – namely, turning my torso to assist as one carer pushed and the other pulled – we could move together smoothly. They placed their palms gently on my shoulders and buttocks and described me as 'helpful'. But, when I appeared to be reluctant in responding, and staff had to lift my legs to turn

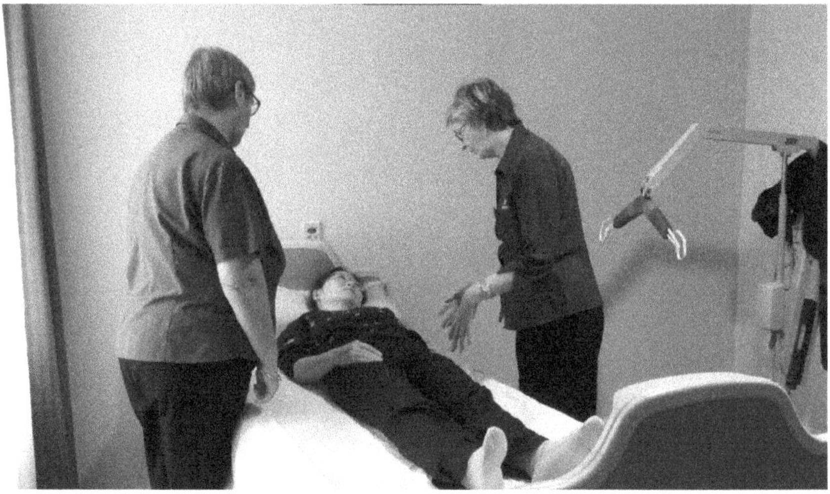

**ILLUSTRATION 0.9.** The ethnographer being assisted by two personal care workers with transferring from bed to chair in 2015. © Angela Zhang.

me, they described the situation as 'difficult', and I could feel discomfort when their fingers gripped me.

I also found that different staff used different manual handling techniques with me, according to their understanding of the resident's bodily condition, as described in the written care plan but also through their long-term experience caring for residents with or without cognitive impairments. One carer might ask me to turn to one side or to lift my leg, whereas her partner, who said that she had most of her shifts in the dementia unit, just silently applied the manual handling procedure, rolling me from side to side. Instead of giving me instructions, she moved me forcibly by pushing, pulling, patting or gripping. 'Residents with dementia don't follow instructions', she explained to me.

Methods used in this study fluctuated as I conducted the fieldwork, and I often expanded beyond research conventions that depend on language and reason. My study of movement needed to include residents with cognitive impairments, who are often excluded from research. This approach departed from conventional methodologies that depend heavily on language, in which participants are expected to produce oral narratives in interviews. The underlying assumption in much qualitative research (even that conducted in nursing homes) is that knowledge about people's experiences, the subjective meanings of what has been lived, can only be gained through verbal communication. But this cannot work for most nursing home residents. Cognitive impairment was very evident at my field study sites, and it meant most residents could not reflect on and articulate their thoughts and feelings. I realized that examining movement was one way that I could study the issues of participants whose concerns could not be articulated, or who articulated their concerns in a fashion that is 'imperceptible' within dominant ways of understanding (Papadopoulos, Stephenson and Tsianos 2008). This study thus offered a different window into how the elderly live their lives in residential care, and at the same time it challenged contemporary perspectives on ageing and dementia.

## Structure of the Ethnographic Study

The book is divided into two sections. The first part focuses on walking by describing how various individual residents experience this important way of moving: it demonstrates that walking is more than an action performed by an isolated individual body; it is an activity entwined with the care provided to the resident by other people and things. Right assemblages of care could create new possibilities for residents to move. Part II extends the analysis on walking to other significant movements. Moving beyond walking as such, to consider sitting, attempted standing and eating, shows the complex and shifting interplay between bodily impairments, material surroundings, aged care discourses and daily practices in the nursing homes. Dying residents live in a kind of tension between the struggle to live and move and the urge to seek relief from their painful and declining bodies.

## Notes

1. The COVID-19 pandemic has led to increased complexity of living and working in an aged care home due to outbreaks and restrictive measures to reduce the spread of COVID-19. My fieldwork was undertaken prior to the pandemic.
2. Final Report of the Royal Commission into Aged Care Quality and Safety (issued on 26 February 2021) revealed that older people in need of care prefer to receive care in their homes (Pagone and Briggs 2021).

# PART I
## Walking

WHAT IS WALKING? IS IT an ability developed in infancy and lost when we age? Is walking, as Ingold (2011: xii) suggests, one modality of moving that is a fundamental mode of being- in-the-world? Such a question may sound strange to ordinary people living their everyday lives, as walking is largely something that we just do without thinking about it; however, Ingold and Vergunst remind us, in their book on the ethnography of walking, that walking is a quintessential feature of what we understand as a human form of life (2008: 1).

It is with this background in mind that I observed a group of residents in aged care. I learned that age-related bodily deterioration may lead to balance and gait impairments that, when combined with attention and cognition deficits, significantly impact on walking, rendering this essential activity of daily life difficult. In this part, we look at the everyday walking of residents to critically examine how that relates to their sense of being-at-home in a nursing home. Studying people who are living the last stages of life, I asked: Is there a connection between continuing to walk and having a sense of home while living in the nursing home setting? For Ingold and Vergunst, 'Just as no definite point marks where we start to walk, so there is no point, on homecoming, at which we come to a stop. ... Barring accident, older people do not, of an instant, stop walking' (2008: 16). Nevertheless, for frail nursing home residents, walking is always a becoming-walking in which tensions between walking and not walking must be continuously negotiated. In chapters 3 and 4, I discuss situations where residents were not assisted to walk as they wished. This paves the way for a fuller discussion on the topic of care in Part II. Care is understood in this study as a dimension of walking. Part I focuses on walking as a way in which residents may feel themselves to be at home in residential care. In Part II, I shift the focus from walking to other activities – for example, standing and eating – to analyse the vital role that care plays in supporting residents to move, and hence to become at home in the nursing homes.

# 1 WATCHING EACH STEP

## Sore Legs and Numb Feet of Mrs Casey

In her ethnography on barefoot running, Warnock describes how barefoot runners experience pleasure as they 'feel the world through their feet', in contrast to shoed runners and walkers, who may still feel the world through their feet but do not experience 'pleasure from the sensation of the ground' (2013: 96).

Our feet are the only area of the body that is in direct contact with the ground as we stand and walk. Walking, running and standing become impossible if our feet are off the ground. Each time we take a step, we preconsciously activate the nerve endings on the soles of the feet. Without conscious attention, we accommodate to our terrain by putting pressure on various parts of the feet and adjusting our position. Whether we are standing up from a chair, walking on a flat pavement or climbing up a slope, similar physiological and neurological processes are involved – we adapt preconsciously by changing how we ground the feet, and the rest of the body responds accordingly. That grounding, or lack thereof, affects our overall posture, movements and stability. Being barefoot or wearing shoes also affects one's grounding and overall experience of running and walking. How we run or walk is also affected by the material environment. Warnock's research reveals how barefoot runners are careful about their choice of trails. Running with bare feet on a rocky road gives pain rather than pleasure. Running on a sun-baked dirt trail may at first feel bouncy and uplifting – every inch of the sole stretches in tune with the rhythmic vibrations we feel. But once that resonance is interrupted by the sharpness of rocks, our steps become uneven, and we soon find ourselves off balance.

While the feet play a crucial role in grounding the person, we are not ordinarily aware of our feet touching the ground while running and walking. 'Walking is an accomplishment of the whole body in motion' (Ingold and Vergunst 2008: 2). We do not experience walking as separate bodily movements, such as putting one foot in front of the other, but as a concerted natural flow of movements. According to Polanyi, all bodily movements involved in walking are in the subsidiary awareness, which is the instrumental attention that gives us a tacit *feel* of our positions and movements in relation to others around us (1958: vii, 91). It gives rise to our experience of walking as 'carefree': little attention is paid to the path on which we walk, or the positions and movements of legs, spine and ankles. People and objects in the environment are incorporated into one's self through the working of subsidiary awareness, which gives the appearance of our natural way of walking.

The other type of awareness that Polanyi describes is focal awareness, which makes walking part of, or supportive to the practical activity in which we are engaged (1958: vii, 91). While I may have a conversation with a friend as we both walk, my focal awareness is on talking and listening. I keep walking without being consciously aware of how my centre of weight is constantly shifting, and my pace adjusts automatically when I need to walk uphill. I do not consciously think about the degree of the incline or the extra effort it takes me to climb it. The subsidiary awareness of moving through place is merged into the focal awareness of holding a conversation while walking. Material things such as the surface of the footpath in relation to my bodily parts become indistinguishable through the coordinated operation of subsidiary awareness. As this brief discussion shows, how my awareness operates is in relation to the presence of many material things in a constantly changing environment. The very fact that I can engage in a conversation while walking shows that my whole body is functioning as one unit. The sensations in the feet, the forward motion of the legs, the rotation of hips and the swinging of arms all contribute to a person's act of walking. What Polanyi conceptualizes, using the terms subsidiary awareness and focal awareness, is how, through the organic synthesis of many conscious and preconscious processes, we relate to the world through sensual incorporation and perceptual objectification – in what is an originary sense of being alive in and through movement (Barbaras 2008).

However, with ageing and bodily decline, the ordinary way of walking can be drastically interrupted, and without grounding the feet, one may lose their footing. Mrs Casey, a nursing home resident with type II diabetes, is an example. Mrs Casey could not feel heat, cold or pain in her feet, even when they were being tightly squeezed into her shoes. The nerves in her lower limbs, including her legs and feet, were damaged due to her long-term diabetes, which led to her condition of 'sensory diabetic neuropathy'. She could only feel a faint sensation in her soles when she walked. The muscles in her feet also did not function properly, because the nerves that make the muscles work were damaged. Consequently, her feet did not align properly. To make her situation worse, the neuropathy caused severe leg pain.

On bad days, she could hardly get out of bed due to sharp pains and feelings of pins and needles in her legs. On these days, Mrs Casey would stay in bed, crouched in the foetal position, moaning.

Mrs Casey's numb, diabetic feet could hardly keep her in touch with the world. Unable to receive the proprioceptive information integral to walking, she struggled to maintain posture, gait and balance while standing or walking. The pain in her legs and the numbness of her feet interrupted the unity of her whole body functioning and changed her prediabetic usual way of walking. Processes usually in her subsidiary awareness – the concerted movements of her feet and legs – were starkly brought into her focal awareness through pain, and the usual flow of movements was broken down into a fractured sequence of slow and separate motions of bodily parts. At times, Mrs Casey was so engulfed by excruciating pain that she could not think about walking.

## Desire to Walk

For a short period after moving into the aged care facility, Mrs Casey avoided walking. For her, walking was painful and risky. She told me that she believed it was 'not the right thing to do' as it could bring on pain, discomfort and a fear of falling. But she soon realized that her nursing home life would be miserable if she stopped walking altogether. Without walking, she was confined to her own room; she rarely saw or talked to anyone other than the staff who delivered meals and pills. Increasingly bored, sedated and isolated, she put on weight and had frequent mood swings. She started to miss the feeling of being able to walk around, have lunch in the dining area and meet people for a chat. The longer she was alone in her room, the stronger was her desire to walk again: she told staff that she wanted to resume walking.

Mrs Casey's urge to resume walking was supported by her doctor and the care management team in the facility. The clinical nurse explained to Mrs Casey that walking is the most effective way to reduce her diabetic pain and potential complications. Recollecting her experience of relearning to walk, Mrs Casey told me that her experience of pain in her legs changed after her conversation with the nurse. She said she used to feel dreadful, with overwhelming pain from severe tissue damage to her legs, and she was faced with the gloomy prospect of having an amputation. She was greatly relieved to know that walking would do no harm to her legs and would help to get her diabetes under control. This new understanding of her bodily condition and situation strengthened Mrs Casey's desire to resume walking. With the belief that her diabetes would be better controlled if she could continue to walk, Mrs Casey relearned how to walk and established a walking routine.

Walking for Mrs Casey was intense and potentially risky, and she often had mixed feelings about doing it. Before each attempt she would fear losing control of her body, falling and injuring herself. Yet, after every walk she did, she felt a sense of peace and accomplishment. Instead of regarding it as a tedious task that she had to do every day, she started to think of walking as a therapy, something she could do to get healthier and feel better in herself. As she continued to walk daily, Mrs Casey started to feel a sense of rightness – that being able to stand on her own two feet and walk again was an outward sign of her improvement. She felt 'right' if she walked and like 'something is not right' if she missed a day whenever her legs hurt. While residents often say, as Mrs Casey said, that they 'can't do much' while confined to residential care, being able to walk and feeling good and right about walking is at the core of how they feel, think and talk about 'feeling at home' in the nursing home.

The first phase of Mrs Casey's relearning to walk involved reconditioning her painful legs. Under the supervision of a physiotherapist's assistant, she stood in front of the handrail in the corridor outside her room and held on to it. With her feet set apart and pressing firmly into the floor, she transferred her weight onto her right foot and slowly lifted her left leg off the floor. She held that position for a few seconds, then she slowly put her left foot back onto the floor. Transferring her weight to her left foot, she slowly lifted her right leg. She tried to disregard initially troubling sensations of pain: 'It's not that bad. It'll get better once I can walk.' Gradually, the pain in her legs became less intense. After her legs became attuned to the concerted movements of the body, Mrs Casey could then shift her focal attention to experiment with taking steps.

With help from the physiotherapist, Mrs Casey learnt to use her sight and conscious attention to monitor the movements of her feet. She carefully placed her left foot on the floor in line with the left wheel of the walker while bending forward from the waist up so she could see her feet moving. Under the normal functioning of our proprioception, the body 'knows' where all its parts are without being able to see them in objective space. However, Mrs Casey needs to see how her feet move in objectified space in order to know how to take the next step. Having learnt to adjust her attentional mode by practising, Mrs Casey could substitute the preconscious proprioceptive perception – sensation from the soles of her feet – with her conscious proprioceptive awareness received through sight. In feeling her way while seeing her feet moving, visual perception of her even strides was synthesized with her proprioceptive perception of balanced posture and gait. In time, although Mrs Casey's walking still looked slow, her improved balance made it seem quite rhythmic and fluent. Achieving better balance and steadiness, she felt 'just right'.

From feeling not right to just right through walking, the process of Mrs Casey relearning to walk is also the process in which someone may be gradually helped to walk again, despite bodily impairments. This phenomenon cannot be explained within the dominant conceptual framework used in aged care for understanding residents' problems with walking. In that discourse, walking is conceptualized as 'ambulation', a modality of mobility, which is the 'ability of older individuals to move within their environment performing functional tasks' (Ouellet and Rush 1996). Within this framework, health professionals and nursing staff tend to understand the walking of residents in terms of their individual capacity to walk and its partial or total loss. There is an assumption that one's functional capacities are bounded within the physical body.

Two central points are key to this conceptualization of capacity as a natural and innate given, both of which I find reductive and problematic. First, the acquisition and/or loss of capacities are thought to be the natural outcome of human development and decline. This invites a direct association between old age and the loss of capacities. Second, taking a reductive approach, the capacity to walk is considered in terms of the respective function of body parts, which is assessed by taking measures of gait, pace and stride. Mobility care, as one category of the institutional practices of aged care service delivery, is organized around this notion of residents' level of mobility. Loss of functional capacities is seen in physiological research as the reduction of physical fitness, including strength, endurance, agility and flexibility (Riebe et al. 2009). Difficulties with walking are ascribed to deteriorating body parts or systems, such as the loss of muscle strength in the lower limbs. The solution to this problem is, therefore, to slow down the loss of functional and physical abilities through exercises targeting failing body parts or systems (Gault and Willems 2013).

In the nursing homes, however, the assessed mobility capacity of a resident is not predictive of whether the resident might be able to move in the course of daily activities. In real-life environments, residents assessed as incapable of walking could, in effect, walk on their own under staff supervision or with the aid of an assistive device. This observation is in line with the findings from Giannouli and colleagues' (2016) research on mobility of older people living in the community. Their research found that mobility performance, as measured in daily living situations, is not simply a matter of functioning within the limits of capacity to move. Rather, that performance reflects how older people are actively exploiting their capacity to be mobile in their everyday lives.

Mrs Casey described a process of 'feeling just right in walking', having increased her confidence in standing up from a reclining chair and being 'less and less worried' every time she set off on her lunchtime walking routine. Mrs Casey attempted to establish a new functional norm – a careful way of walking – by navigating the limitations caused by her diabetes.

In relearning to walk, Mrs Casey was deploying her remaining capacities of attention and response. Practising exercises, such as sit–stand with handrail, and wall push-ups, meant that her whole body could be in motion despite its local impairments. Through individualized scheduled exercises, Mrs Casey worked on her core muscles, back, butt and hips, to improve her balance and mobility. In this sense, the sore legs and numb feet of Mrs Casey became the central motivation in her relearning to walk, thus demonstrating that bodies are not fragmented collections of parts but operate as multiplicities that hang together in various forms of coordination. In a sector where the dominant discourse is about decline, disability and impairment, relearning skills and expanding the body's capacities are often seen as unrealistic, if not entirely unthinkable. But, as demonstrated by Mrs Casey's deliberative and adaptive response to bodily decline, relearning to walk was indeed made possible. Relearning a movement is, in effect, a matter of growth, expanding one's capacity into a new bodily condition so that the person can continue to move.

## Walking Aid: The Best Walking Companion

The process of Mrs Casey relearning to walk also involved assistance from other material things and persons. Her 'wheelie walker' played a pivotal role in helping her to eventually place one foot firmly in front of the other. Mrs Casey was initially assessed by the physiotherapist as needing '1-staff physical assistance with transfers and locomotion', which meant she was prescribed the help of one personal care worker to provide support, either by holding her back or arm, when getting out of bed, standing up from a chair or walking. As Mrs Casey is heavily built and overweight, it did not take long for her and the staff to realize that one care worker could not safely help her with transfers and walking. But Mrs Casey came to dislike the required physical contact from carers, such as a hand on her lower back, which gave her an uneasy feeling and distracted her from walking. The physiotherapist subsequently prescribed a 4-wheeled walker to assist Mrs Casey with her walking. A 4-wheeled walker is designed for users who can walk reasonably well but would benefit from extra support over longer distances. However, in the case of Mrs Casey, the support from her walker was crucial. 'You can't walk without your best friend, Mrs Casey!'

staff would often joke in reference to her walker. The word 'right' was frequently used by staff to refer to situations, such as these, when residents were observed to be able to move. They saw that the walker provided the right type and amount of assistance, and it was hailed as 'just right for Mrs Casey'.

But it could take time for residents to feel their walking aid was the right fit for them. According to Mrs Casey, the walker felt strange when she first took hold of it. Its plastic handlebars were cold to touch. Its wheels were either too fast or too slow in response to her handling. 'I didn't feel it would suit me when I first started,' Mrs Casey said. Yet, as time went on, she experimented with the walker to make it fit her style of movement better. First she lowered the handlebars so she could push using her hands, and then later raised the handlebars to try pushing with her elbows. She would push it to stand up, pull it to sit down or lean on it to take a breath.

With time and practice, as staff commented, the walker increasingly fitted the bill, aiding Mrs Casey's posture, gait and balance. In observing that Mrs Casey was able to walk safely with the aid of the walker, staff documented in 'progress notes' that this solution was 'right' for Mrs Casey.

The right assistive technology, of course, differs from person to person. An aid is something that has to fit the user's body, and each body is unique. For Mrs Casey, this fit was demonstrated in several ways. First, in contrast to standard usage, which requires the person to hold the frame at a comfortable position in front of the body, usually with a 15 to 30 degree bend at the elbow to facilitate standing in an upright position, Mrs Casey did not hold the handlebars with her hands, nor did she take an upright posture. Instead, she bent herself forward from the waist up, leaning on the walker using her elbows. She bent forward heavily on her walker with her upper body positioned at a roughly 100 degree angle. The centre of gravity was therefore not in the base of the walker or in any part of her body: it was somewhere in between Mrs Casey and the walker. This is because the only way could she move her feet was when part of her body weight was transferred onto the walker. The walking aid thus provided both additional support and a wider centre of gravity. Second, Mrs Casey directed her body weight through her elbows to the walking aid, meaning there was less impact on, and lower static forces passing through, her arthritic knees and ankles. Thus the walking aid, combined with her supporting arms, could compensate for weaker muscles and joints of the spine, pelvis and legs and generate the dynamic forces needed for walking.

Once she felt the walker fitted her, the way that it aided her required no conscious attention. She did not look down at either the walker or the positions of her elbows as she pushed the walker forward. Her elbows rested easily on the handlebars of the walker. When I once tried the same posture, my body tensed up and I had to concentrate hard to not lose my balance. My neck hurt when I looked up from this much lower position; my back complained from being bent over at a right angle – to me, it was an awkward and nerve-wracking posture. Yet, the walker came to suit Mrs Casey like a handy hammer ready-to-hand – tacit knowing through touch.

In contrast to healthy adults, the walking of residents often involved the use of an aid device such as the wheelie walker or assistance from staff. Walking was therefore not a matter of moving alone but moving alongside another person or thing, which then calls for the *attunement* or *synergy* described by Ingold (2011: 17). Using the example of a person sawing through a plank of wood, he says that sawing, a rhythmic activity requiring manual dexterity, involves a kind of attunement that calls for intense concentration. Ingold explains that the concentration '… is that of a consciousness that is not confined within the head of the practitioner but reaches out into the environment along multiple pathways of sensory participation' to 'bring into phase an ensemble of concurrent movements, both within and beyond the body' (2011: 18). In resting her elbows on the handlebars and aligning her feet with its wheels, Mrs Casey and her walker moved into concordance.

Following a walking routine may similarly become a ritual-like performance that brings the person into a particular state of being. In a different example, after personally experiencing the Warlpiri ceremony in central Australia, Jackson was convinced that:

> … a sense of home is grounded less in a place per se than in the activity that goes on in a place … concentrated activity is experienced as a quickened relationship between oneself and whatever one works upon. The object comes to embody the life of the worker. This means that before Warlpiri recognize a metaphorical fusion between person and place, this fusion is felt in bodily praxis. (M. Jackson 1995: 148)

What is described as fusion between person and place through ceremonial dancing in Jackson's case becomes a synergy of practitioner, tool and material in Ingold's skilled sawing activity.

As the descriptions demonstrate, in relearning to walk, Mrs Casey could *attune* to her declining body and meanwhile *connect* with the right things (e.g. a suitable walking aid) and persons (attending staff members) to establish *adaptive* new forms of walking. To further illustrate Mrs Casey's walking as a way of feeling 'right at home' in the nursing home, the next section describes how she could manage to walk safely – taking each step with care – relating to her surroundings with sensibility and responsiveness.

## Watching Each Step

As we have seen, Mrs Casey walked in a unique manner, bending herself forward from the waist up and leaning onto the walker using her elbows. There is a special reason for this gait: it was crucial for her to see her own feet moving to ensure she lowered each foot to the floor in turn and that its position was correct in relation to the position of her walker. She would not have been able to lift her other foot and swing it forward if the positioning of the supporting foot did not look right. 'I must watch every step of mine,' Mrs Casey once told me, explaining how she managed to walk safely. Unlike for able-bodied healthy adults, walking becomes a highly concentrated activity for residents like Mrs Casey. This modality of residents' walking can be described as 'careful' – taking each step very slowly – so that they will not trip over, lose balance and potentially have a fall. I will go into more detail to illustrate how Mrs Casey could feel just right and retain a sense of control while walking safely.

Mrs Casey was very focused once she started walking. She did not look ahead or around but just down at her own moving feet. She kept surprisingly steady with each step, although progress was painfully slow. After about four steps, she might stop walking and look around. This was the only time that she responded to people around her. While actually walking, she simply ignored anyone who passed by and said 'Hello!' to her. I once asked whether she needed some help when I met her in the foyer. She paid no attention to me until she came to a full stop. She turned her head to the side, to where I was standing, and looked up: 'No, leave me alone. It's better to let me do it,' she answered and slowly resumed her walking. Annie, a veteran care worker, later advised me not to talk to Mrs Casey while she was fully engaged in her walking: 'Better leave her to concentrate on her walking. When they age, they cannot cope with more than one task. Mrs Casey would feel overwhelmed to have a conversation with you while walking.'

After having observed Mrs Casey walking along the corridors for a few months, I came to a deeper understanding of her unique way of walking. Her walking pattern included a sequence of slow-motion movements of her feet, a rhythm of a four-four beat (four steady strides) then rest (stop to look around), and the style was marked by an arched posture over her walker and a noticeable rotation of her hips. Unlike the ordinary way of walking, Mrs Casey had to maintain an intensified focal attentiveness, and this led to a loss of fluency in her movements. Walking carefully meant paying particular attention to each step she took: any interference might have disrupted her rhythm of walking.

There are three key features of Mrs Casey's careful walking to consider. First, she largely relied on visual perception to monitor the position of her feet and to control the movement of her legs. Her close watching of every movement of her feet suggests that there are perceptual processes involved, including comparison of positions, judgement on distance and decisions on fine-tuning the movements. Second, it took all of Mrs Casey's visual concentration to control her movements as she walked. A single, simple motor activity, like walking on a carpeted floor, was all she could manage at one time. Multitasking, such as talking while walking, would affect her concentration and lead to loss of control over her movements. Finally, such a careful way of walking is necessarily time- and energy-consuming. Her speed was slow. The fact that the movements of lifting up and swinging of her lower limbs had to be consciously monitored and controlled slowed each step down. She needed to stop after every four steps to regain her energy. The distance she walked (from her room to the dining area) was short, and the frequency (twice a day) low because of the mental effort and energy expended.

As a kinaesthetic form of activity, walking is often experienced by healthy able-bodied adults as fluent and effortless. Bodies move on their own with little conscious awareness. Yet, walking became an intense activity for Mrs Casey. She had to make an extraordinary effort to accomplish a daily walking routine. This leads to the question that is key to the investigation and argument of this book: namely, how could the activity of walking enable a sense of feeling at home if it involved so much effort? Seeking answers to this question, the next section considers the walking routine of Mrs Casey as a sensory extension. Through this, she became familiar with the nursing home environment and then, eventually, step by step, she came to feel at home there.

## Becoming-at-Home in a Walking Routine

Routines reflect residents' individual concerns, interests and preferences. How well elderly residents can adjust to an institutional way of life and inhabit the nursing home environment is affected by the extent to which they are supported to establish and follow everyday personal routines. Previous research on residents establishing daily routines in a Hong Kong nursing home found that routine is neither the exact same activity that one experienced before, nor does it refer to a completely different form of activity that bears no relation to past experience. Newly admitted nursing home residents in a Hong Kong care facility were found to attempt to 'fit in by repatterning their lifestyles and daily routines as much as they could' (Lee, Woo and Mackenzie 2002: 671). Re-creating home in the nursing home, or 'regaining normality', to use Lee's term, is a process of reformation in which residents actively fit previous home habits and routines into the nursing home environment so that new routine practices emerge.

My observations in the care facilities in Adelaide reveal that to fit home habits and routines into the nursing home environment residents undergo a process of *in-habiting* – entering continuous and uncertain processes of 'doing undergoing', which might be described as 'the evanescent reality of movement' (Sheets-Johnstone 2011: 126). Establishing a walking routine, as the example of Mrs Casey shows, involves movements that are not merely repetitions but also require numerous circumstantial modifications. For anyone who is learning or relearning to walk, the process involves a lot of repetitive practice, which in itself establishes 'habit' as a kind of movement in which we and those who move with us, and to whom we relate, will 'in-habit together' in the world (Dewey 2015). Adolph and colleagues' (2012) research details the immense amount of practice involved in learning to walk: on average, 12- to 19-month-old toddlers took 2,368 steps and fell 17 times per hour. Despite the obvious differences between infants learning to walk and elderly residents relearning to walk, they share the need for repetitive practice. Both the very young and the very old experience bodily changes in and through the movements they make and the postures they adopt. Learning or relearning a movement takes place in the environments that are at once physical and sociocultural. Infants not only grow into walking; they grow into the expected ways of walking, which are shaped by the material things that they walk upon, through and with, as well as the persons with whom they walk alongside (Adolph et al. 2012). Relearning a movement is not only about the particular movement per se. While walking becomes an everyday routine activity, selected material things and acquainted places are regularly and consistently incorporated into the self through sensory extension (Dennis 2007). In relearning to walk, Mrs Casey reconfigured her bodily capacities to see and feel, push and pull, attend to and respond towards the material things and persons encountered in her day-to-day life. Over a period of more than two years, Mrs Casey always lived in the same room, but by regularly walking, she became engaged with life beyond her own four walls. It is the keeping up of routine activities that matters to people, as Latimer and Munro (2009) argue, because it brings about a regular, mundane affirmation of what and who it is that they care for. Mrs Casey cared to keep in touch with her surroundings through daily walking.

It is important to note that while residents' daily walking is regarded as an established routine that can be embedded and repeated, it is in effect an open-ended improvising process: '... guided by the past but not determined by it; heading into a future that is essentially unforeseeable' (Ingold and Hallam 2007: 11). To familiarize herself with every inch of the corridors linking her room to the dining area, Mrs Casey was always careful to observe her surroundings. She stopped to watch or ask if she saw any changes: an obstacle on the floor, a sharp turn around the corner or a new piece of furniture. Mrs Casey knew that, if she happened to step on a raised bit of carpet, she would not be able to adjust her posture to stabilize herself and she would trip and fall over. Walking was thus, for Mrs Casey, a process of exploiting the dynamics and potentials of staying upright. Only by a process of repeating and improvising could she maintain a sense of control while walking in and through her surroundings.

Over time, Mrs Casey became woven into what Ingold (2011) describes as meshwork – in this case, the organic interconnectedness of the nursing home – and she grew to know her surroundings intimately. She would naturally turn to the other side of the corridor to avoid the lump in the carpet. She stopped to watch for oncoming traffic before making a turn at the sharp corner. The sensory and tangible properties of the material things around her, like the red colours of the carpet and the sheen of the polished timber floor, became attuned to her movements through her perception and proprioception. Her careful way of walking became part and parcel of her sense of home, providing a sense of permanence and security in a dynamically unpredictable world. For residents like Mrs Casey, a personal walking routine enabled a processual 'becoming-at-home' in the nursing home.

## Achieving a Balance: The Becoming of a Walking Routine

Jackson wrote that being is 'living the tension between acting on one's own will and being acted upon by others to which one has no control' (2002: 14). In Jackson's theorization on home, being able to act autonomously plays a central role in having a sense of control and connectedness, creating a sense of being-at-home-in-the-world. For Rapport, a social ethics of care for elderly people needs to focus on 'caring that their autonomy is not infringed' (2018: 256). He draws on Jackson's notion of home to suggest that elderly people may not be able to have a sense of home while experiencing the tension between being autonomous and being controlled by others. He points out that, as long as their lives are being managed by other people, aged residents are to some extent being prevented from exercising their free will.

Researchers find that the institutional routine practices of care, when strictly followed, do constrain the people who live there. As an exercise of institutional regulatory power, routine care practices 'are driven more by a desire for organizational efficiency than the comfort of residents' (Bland 2003: 187). Bland's research highlights the seemingly all-powerful control of the institution over its members, residents and staff alike, who are expected to be passive. While Vesperi (1983) considers the paternalistic management of older people's lives as the outcome of cultural influence, Gubrium (1975) points to the structural barrier between those who manage the lives of the patients and those who are managed. The administrators who make decisions for the patients often do not understand the complexity of care processes from the perspectives of patients and caregivers. A focus on the soft yet imposing power of the institution highlights how elderly residents usually have little control over the ways in which they are cared for.

Other researchers have investigated residents' adaptive efforts while living within the constraints of institutional life. Kayser-Jones (1981) found that the adaptive capacity of residents was shown in their efforts to reciprocate with staff in different ways, including being compliant with staff demands. Harnett's (2010) research also demonstrated how residents in a Swedish nursing home attempted to garner back some small vestige of power within the constraints of the institution. To exert subtle influence on inflexible institutional routines, residents tried ploys, such as asking staff for a change of bedtime, in an attempt to carve out some autonomy or express personal preferences in their everyday lives.

In contrast to research findings that residents had little control over their daily activities, Lovatt (2018) found that some residents demonstrated their control of, and sense of belonging to the institution through the material furnishing of their rooms. Using data collected through participant observation and in-depth interviews in an English nursing home, Lovatt shows that residents cultivated a sense of home in their individual rooms by establishing regular practices, routines and interactions with their material surroundings. Routine activities such as cleaning and hosting visitors, without any staff participation, became their *own practices* of 'doing home'. Lovatt maintains that in this way residents do exert choice, or what can be thought of as 'acting', in Jackson's framework. In showing that residents make choices, or act with a sense of control, Lovatt depicts these lives as far from constrained.

My own observations in the nursing homes revealed the nuances of routine practices as multiplicities – becomings of daily activities that could not be understood in terms of any singular notion of control. I found that the ways in which Mrs Casey could relearn to walk, establish and follow a walking routine was not an example of walking as simply doing (for oneself) *or* being done (by others), but rather, as Rapport (2018) argues, it struck a balance between engagement and inclusion on the one hand, and a preservation of autonomy and personal sovereignty on the other. The term 'balance' is used in Rapport's social ethics of care to describe an appropriate proportionality to autonomy and inclusion. In other words, a balance must be achieved in the processes of caring, which will be different for every bodily condition and situation.

For residents with physical impairments but cognitive competence, like Mrs Casey, the innermost drive to move manifests itself in activities involving cognition including choosing to relearn to walk rather than sitting in a wheelchair, taking efforts to relearn to walk and to establish and follow a daily walking routine. Once Mrs Casey had this initiative, she was strategic about developing her walking routine. After relearning the skills to walk safely with her walker, she slowly increased her walking distance and negotiated between routes that were easy to navigate and those encumbered by a flow of trolleys, wheelchairs and staff rushing from place to place. Gradually, as she came to be familiar with the environment, she became more at ease with her careful walking. She took care to always walk at the same time, once before lunch and a second time after lunch, and took the same route: from her room to the dining area and back. From taking that first step to following a daily walking routine, Mrs Casey was taking control of her own life course as well as her own movements.

Nevertheless, what staff think of as a resident's *personal* routine, such as the walking routine of Mrs Casey, is not only governed by the resident's own choices and efforts. Walking is never just a matter of resident choice. Permission to walk is contingent on multiple factors. Mrs Casey did not act solely according to her own choice, free of external influence and control. Her decision to relearn to walk and follow a daily walking routine had to be made in consultation with the care management team in the facility. Being capable of verbal communication and establishing relationships with staff was important for Mrs Casey; it meant she could strategically incorporate a walking routine into her care plan so that it could then be integrated into staff delivery of care. In establishing a walking routine, Mrs Casey was anticipating and thinking through how and when staff could be involved, so that staff assistance could be prescheduled. As a routine part of care, staff usually came to Mrs Casey at a quarter to twelve, stood her walker in front of her, and got her ready for the walk to the dining area for lunch, which was served at twelve o'clock. The efforts of Mrs Casey, the presence and assistance of staff and the involvement of her walker in her transfers all together achieved a balance. It was this balance that enabled Mrs Casey to follow her walking routine and feel more at home in the nursing home.

In aged care facilities in Australia, the resident care plan that is created on admission to a nursing home is mostly made after consultation with the resident and their significant others to reflect their own interests and preferences. As time goes by, the daily activities that are carried out become routinized into a *habit* for both residents and staff through repetitive practice. The term 'habit' is used here in the sense that Ingold (2017) has developed from Dewey's (2015) notion of habit to refer to a forwarding and open-ended process of 'doing undergoing'. In considering habit as process, Ingold emphasizes the uncertainty, potentiality and probability involved in habitual engagements. This opens the possibilities of considering routine practices not through the notion of control but of *balance*. With the notion of balance, one's own efforts and others' engagements can be 'rightly' incorporated into residents' walking and consequent feelings of being 'all right' and 'at home'. Thus, Mrs Casey's daily walking can be understood as demonstrating how a simple routine can serve as a reference point for shared work and joint efforts of care, combining flows of movements of residents, walking aids and staff into an assemblage that supports Mrs Casey and those like her to create a sense of being-at-home in the nursing home.

# 2 BEYOND WANDERING

## Mrs Sage: The Wandering Lady

Unlike residents with cognitive competence, like Mrs Casey, who could feel right at home in and through walking by being attentive, learning to watch each step and following a walking routine, residents with severe cognitive impairments, like Mrs Sage, lived at home in the nursing home in a very different way.

Everyone in the dementia care unit knew Mrs Sage, not always by name but rather as 'the wandering lady'. I first met Mrs Sage when I followed Mike, a registered nurse, on his last round of the 'day checks' in the two secure dementia units that he supervises. She walked towards us. At first sight, I was stunned by her skeletal figure, with eyes that seemed disproportionately large against her hollowed face. She seemed to look towards us, yet her face was expressionless. As we approached her, she seized the handrail with both hands. They were bony, criss-crossed with blue veins, the fingers crooked and the joints visibly red and swollen. Mike silently stood aside, and she carried on walking. I could see he looked concerned as he watched the elderly woman pass by and move unsteadily to the end of the corridor. This was not Mike's usual response to a resident: ordinarily he would stop a few steps away and lower his six-foot frame to greet residents face to face, cheerfully with a grin. 'Who is she?' I asked. 'Mrs Sage', Mike answered quietly. After spending a few days in the unit, I came to realize that how Mike gave way to this resident was typical among the staff. As she walks around, they clear a passageway for her. No one says anything to her, and she talks to no one.

Staff repeatedly referred to Mrs Sage's walking as 'wandering', and this was constructed as an unfortunate kind of movement that was both excessive and aimless. 'She gets started as soon as her feet touch the floor. She is forever on her run from morning to night', Annie, a veteran carer, told me. Indeed, Mrs Sage did seem to be unstoppable once she started walking. Without a fixed course or goal, no definite starting and ending points, the walking path of Mrs Sage was a puzzle to onlookers. More like a mesh of threads than a straight line from A to B, her constant zig-zag paths along the corridors were punctuated by predictable stops at locked doors or resting places where she could hold on to a handrail or a piece of furniture.

In contrast to the purposeful walking exhibited by Mrs Casey, Mrs Sage appeared to roam aimlessly along the corridors of the nursing home, loping around with jerky steps and bumping into laundry or food trolleys. She would push her way through groups of people chatting in the lounge or career into sofas, chairs or dining tables. Such haphazard movement among fragile residents in communal areas was potentially disruptive to staff, other residents and visitors. Consequently, her presence often stirred up a wave of shouts and scolding from other residents. One day there was an incident when she grabbed onto Mrs Hayley, who was sitting on a couch in the lounge, and threw her arms around the elderly woman's neck. Mrs Hayley's daughter, Isabella, happened to be visiting and saw this incident.

'Does she know what she is doing?' exclaimed Isabella, angrily. Isabella called Sharon, the registered nurse on duty, to the scene. She described what had happened to Sharon and referred to the incident as 'harassment'. Sharon calmly replied: 'Probably not. She is not quite herself now. Her dementia has got worse.' Pointing her index finger to her own head, Sharon added: 'Her mind has gone.' Dismissing Isabella's suggestion that Mrs Sage had purposely hurtled into Mrs Hayley, Sharon attributed Mrs Sage's behaviour to her 'loss of mind and self', shorthand for cognitive impairments and personality changes, conceived in biomedicine as some of the adverse outcomes of dementia.

'What on earth happens to people when they get dementia? She must be crazy', said Isabella, sounding less angry but still confused. Sharon explained: 'Well, Mrs Sage can't talk. She can't tell us what she wants or why. Maybe she is bored, maybe she has no control over what she does. Whatever the causes are, it's her dementia to blame, not her.' Here Sharon was emphasizing the fact that Mrs Sage could not express herself because of her dementia. According to Sharon, dementia had taken complete control over Mrs Sage, affecting her walking and how she responded towards others. She implied: how could anyone blame this mute and lost elderly lady for being incapable of controlling her own movements?

After a pause, Sharon added: 'She can still walk though. We can't stop her from walking unless she is a danger to other residents. If you decide to lodge a complaint, I will contact Mrs Sage's doctor. He may agree to prescribe some medication to restrain Mrs Sage from walking.' 'No, that's not what I want at all.' Now Isabella looked horrified. 'There is no point in blaming her for something she has no control over. After all, Mum seems okay.' She sighed, shook her head and left.

Staff working in the secure dementia unit always defended Mrs Sage from the push-backs and criticisms from residents, and against occasional complaints from families; however, they did regard her walking as a menace – frightening to other residents, detrimental to her own health and disruptive to care delivery. They tried different strategies, such as getting Mrs Sage to sit down with a cup of tea and a sandwich, but Mrs Sage showed no interest in sitting down or eating. She began rapidly losing weight and was prescribed a formula drink with added nutrition. In actual fact, the carers could only feed her with meals and drinks when they could catch hold of her in passing. Once I observed that Mrs Sage even kept marching on the spot while being fed and would walk away with a mouthful of minced beef if not held still by others. Feeding her required two staff, one to hold her still and another to feed her. Since extra staff time and effort were needed to serve her meals and drinks, feeding Mrs Sage could not be integrated into the facility's routine of serving meals. Extra assistance was also required to keep Mrs Sage safe from injuring herself, and she was considered at high risk of falls because of her constant walking. It worried the carers when they saw her clutching the handrails in the hallways and breathing heavily, clearly exhausted from her walking.

As shown in her attempt to protect Mrs Sage, Sharon, the registered nurse, used the neuropathological model of dementia to interpret Mrs Sage's behaviour. The walking was recorded in Mrs Sage's progress notes as 'wandering behaviour'. In biomedical research, constructing residents' walking as 'wandering' classes such movement as a pathological behaviour. This reductionist model focuses on individual movements that are decontextualized from the broader social, relational and material worlds in which residents are embedded. Bipedal movements are classified as 'lapping', 'pacing' or 'loping', signifying the type of locomotion behaviour associated with the brain damage that is characteristic of dementia and that is medically conceptualized as 'wandering' (Algase et al. 2007). It is therefore classed as one of the behavioural and psychological symptoms of dementia.

Correlation between seemingly irrational ways of walking and the brain damage caused by a neuropathological condition, such as Alzheimer's disease, is well established in biomedical discourse and often used as an interpretative framework by nursing home staff. During one Dementia Dynamics (person-centred care) training session, a picture of the diseased brain, taken in autopsy, was shown side by side with a picture of a normal brain, to demonstrate the stark differences between them. The message is clear and biomedically legitimated: residents with dementia can no longer sense, perceive, think and communicate as normal people do. Residents like Mrs Sage are living as altered beings in their own life world – unable to express themselves or control how they relate to others. 'There are big holes in her brain. Nothing you can do about it,' said one carer, as they discussed Mrs Sage with a hopeless expression.

Suffering such a 'loss of mind and self', as Sharon described it to Isabella, Mrs Sage seemed like a being completely cut off from her surroundings. But did this have to be the case? Could residents with cognitive impairments, like Mrs Sage, re-create a sense of connectedness with other material things and persons? How did her excessive walking impact on her experiences of other people and material things in the nursing home? Before I turn to my thick description of Mrs Sage's walking, let's go a little deeper into our understanding of the cognitive impairments that Mrs Sage suffers. First, I would like to refer to Rapport's (2018) concept of 'personal preserve', which is part of his social ethics of care framework. This explains the linkages between personal preserve (in which cognitive abilities are central), individual autonomy and a sense of being-at-home-in-the-world that will help us make sense of the case of Mrs Sage and others with similar cognitive impairments.

## Personal Preserve: What Is Left of Mrs Sage?

Rapport's social ethics of care focuses on the preservation of the individual's 'personal preserve', which he defines as 'a description of individual consciousness as a thing apart, distinct from the world around it' (2018: 254). At the core of his notion of personal preserve is 'the free expressions of a mature consciousness' in the form of first-person point of view, personal sensorium, individual mind and purposeful actions shaping one's life course. The term 'personal preserve' relates to a person's embodied consciousness, which is the decisive centre of attention, perception and action. Focusing on the individualization of self, Rapport suggests the notion that autonomy originates from a decisive centre – the individual consciousness.

According to Rapport, 'personal preserve' is not only the part of us that constitutes individuality and autonomy; it also contributes to our sense of being-at-home-in-the-world by striking a balance between anonymity and autonomy and overcoming the tension between being for oneself and being for others. Speaking from the assumption that any conscious individual should be autonomous, Rapport proposes a general form of ethical care that pertains to individuals across all age groups and stages of life. For the elderly, Rapport insists that the same ethics of care apply 'so far as possible, and for as long as possible' (2018: 255). What goes without saying is that the 'possible' stops when the individual's personal preserve is no more or it becomes impossible to protect and preserve. In short, personal preserve, conceived as the embodied consciousness making a person an autonomous individual, is in danger of gradual loss in old age and so, in turn, is the older person's individuality, autonomy and sense of being-at-home.

Rapport sees the embodied consciousness as a defining feature of being with others in the world, and the person–other relatedness represents the direct connection of the self to surrounding objects. The content of consciousness can be the 'self', the one who experiences, or the 'other', something or someone external to the one who experiences. The directedness of consciousness from self to other things and people is captured in the concept of intentionality. Two modalities of intentionality, 'self-referential' (directed towards self) and 'other-oriented' (directed towards the other), structure experience at the conscious level. In self-reflection and direct observation, subjective experience can be thought of and understood using these concepts.

Yet, it is hypothesized in biomedical research that patients with Alzheimer's disease lose the ability to see themselves from a third-person perspective (Salmon et al. 2005). This leads to an altered experience of being conscious of self, for example, in the areas of self-referential intentionality and body image. An ethnographic vignette illustrates this disjuncture. One day, I chanced to observe Mrs Sage attending a hairdressing appointment. At the salon, staff assisted Mrs Sage to sit in a chair. One carer held both her hands down while the hairdresser quickly set about cutting her hair. When the hairdresser finished her last touches, the carer sat Mrs Sage in a wheelchair and took her in front of a mirror. The carer then made a gesture inviting Mrs Sage to look at her own image in the mirror. As if she was suddenly seized, Mrs Sage thrust herself up from the wheelchair with an intense look on her face. Fixated and motionless, she gazed at the image of herself in the mirror for a few seconds. She then collapsed into the wheelchair as if she could no longer hold herself together. Was she startled or surprised? How Mrs Sage responded to her own image in the mirror was clearly different from that of people with ordinary cognitive functioning.

With impaired self-referential intentionality, the boundaries between oneself and others appear blurred, which affects how one can interact with the world around. Mrs Sage could no longer construct will–be/self–other relationships to guide her actions. She also had no insight into her own wandering, or relationships with others. In the example of her physical contact with Mrs Hayley, Mrs Sage was not only incapable of planning a deliberate attack on Mrs Hayley, but it also raises a question about whether Mrs Sage even understood the meaning of such contact or the reactions it might draw from other people. Furthermore, she would not even be able to recall the incident once she had turned around and left.

Biomedical research suggests that almost all cognitive functions of patients in the later stages of Alzheimer's disease are severely impaired (Förstl and Kurz 1999). For Mrs Sage, her abilities for logical reasoning, planning and organizing had long disappeared. Incapable of relating to others through symbolic representation in any form, she became highly distractible by stimuli and unable to focus on any purposive activity. Unlike Mrs Casey, Mrs Sage was incapable of being attentional, reflective and careful. Moreover, she could no longer form short-term memories, and her longer-term autobiographical memory was for the most part lost. She no longer knew who she was, or had been, and could not recognize her family members and friends.

Mrs Sage is also completely mute and does not respond to verbal language, which restricts her from interpersonal communication. Non-verbal communication was also difficult as Mrs Sage could no longer recognize a material object by its name or symbol. The 'meanings' of material things and beings were no longer suggested to her by their symbolic features. Rather, she made sense of them through immediate and spontaneous encounters with them in and through sensory incorporation and movement. In other words, Mrs Sage could not know a thing by its symbolic representation or think through ideas that might represent things or events. Rather, Mrs Sage only became aware of other material things and beings when she caught sight of them, or heard them, or touched them. Severe cognitive impairments had brought devastating consequences in the everyday life of Mrs Sage: she could not be left alone without fear of injury. Consequently, Mrs Sage relied on staff assistance for all activities of daily living, including eating, drinking, washing and grooming.

The example of Mrs Sage shows that her cognitive impairments had destroyed the agentive 'free expressions of a mature consciousness', as Rapport puts it, in the form of memory, attention, concentration, perception, self-reflection and decision-making. With cognitive faculties impaired to this extent, what was left of the 'personal preserve' of Mrs Sage? On the surface, she seemed to have lost the personal preserve that, according to Rapport, makes us autonomous individuals. But, before we make that assumption, let's ask the question: does being autonomous simply refer to what we express in speech, thought or action? Don't we first move around, making sense of whatever is next to us, before we can possibly engage ourselves in conscious cognitive activities such as contemplation, communication and interaction? Setting Rapport's notion of personal preserve to one side for now, I will next turn to Ingold's examination of the activity of walking.

## Being Alive in Moving through the World

In his influential book *Being Alive*, Tim Ingold (2011) speculated that being alive is a process of moving, knowing and describing. He wrote:

> [To] move, to know, and to describe are not separate operations that follow one another in series, but rather parallel facets of the same process – that of life itself. It is by moving that we know, and it is by moving, too, that we describe. It is absurd to ask, for example, whether ordinary walking is a way of moving, knowing or describing. It is all three at once. ... Philosophers have meditated at length on the condition of being-in-the-world. Moving, knowing and describing, however, call for more than being *in*, or immersion. They call for observation. A being that moves, knows and describes must be observant. Being observant means being alive *to* the world. (Ingold 2011: xii; italics original)

In this excerpt, Ingold makes distinctions between being-*in*-the-world – moving without observing and describing – and being-*to*-the-world – being observant while moving. He asserts that being observant is characteristic of what he calls 'the ordinary way of walking'. Moving, knowing and describing are three integral facets of the same process of life itself. Life is more than being *in* among others without knowing and describing them. While being immersive means being-*in*-the-world; being observant is being-*to*-the-world.

Ingold's distinctions between the two modes of being is useful in our understanding of the various and altered ways of residents' walking. But before I go further to analyse residents' walking, I need first draw on Rapport and Dawson's (1998) work on perception to tease out the terms 'observing' and 'describing'. Rapport and Dawson assert that: 'To conceive relationships (and so create things) is to move or cause to move things relative to the point of perception (the brain) or relative to other things within the field of perception' (1998: 19–20). According to that definition, perceiving (observing) is to separate a 'thing' from 'others' in relation to 'self' so that meaning can be formed and attached to the 'thing' (describing) according to its relationship to itself and others. Thus, 'subject and object, perceiver and perceived are intrinsically connected' (Rapport and Dawson 1998: 20). Rapport and Dawson conclude that movement is fundamental to the creation of thingness, of self and others, and its interconnectedness. So the word 'movement' can be used to refer to the experiences of observing and describing: searching for meanings by relating the other to self while differentiating both from the surroundings in a perceptual world. The experience of observing and describing thus always involves an awareness of self and the self–other relationship; it can construct a world of relationships between the self and other material things or persons. Movement in this sense is by nature perceptual and cognitive, leading to the creation of images, symbols, thoughts, ideas and speech.

This leads to the realization that, for Ingold, walking is not simply about physically travelling over a distance but is more to do with perceiving, knowing and understanding the person–other–world relationships as one moves through the world among others. Holding an idea of a physical place in mind and walking towards it, as a goal, summarizes how people move through their environments: they do so according to their understanding of their own relationship to other material things and beings. In the example of Mrs Casey, the dining area where she usually went for her lunch was the destination of her daily walking. So the perceived person–other relationship can be expressed as a goal-oriented activity in linguistic form: 'Mrs Casey usually goes to the dining area for lunch.' In a metaphorical sense, while a goal for the movement is constructed in the mind in a cognitive process, the body that then moves could be described as a minded body. Walking towards a goal can be understood as a process in which heterogeneous bodies, whether physiological, psychological or social, are blended through the processes of sensing, moving and thinking, into assemblages. Walking, as an activity of moving through the world among others, thus becomes an accomplishment of the whole body in motion (Ingold and Vergunst 2008). This sense of a kind of bodily synthesis is what people experience every day. They experience walking as a coherent process of concerted movements, not as parallel facets or bodily processes. Like ordinary people in similar situations, Mrs Casey just routinely walked to have lunch, without wondering where or why she was going. A sense of control over her own walking came from a productive process of bodily synthesis in which she felt 'just right'.

The experience of being oneself comes from our experience of what has been termed 'psychological continuity and connectedness' (Parfit 1984: 206). We assume that we are the same person across time. We are the author of our thoughts and actions, and we are distinct from our environment. We have the preconscious sensation of mental, emotional and bodily unity, which together forms the experience of being oneself. What is consciously experienced as psychological continuity and connectedness thus involves the synthesis of many preconscious bodily processes of desiring-production (Deleuze and Guattari 1977).

However, for residents with cognitive impairments, like Mrs Sage, syntheses on the perceptual and reflective levels are damaged. Mrs Sage could no longer recognize a material object by its name or symbol. Rather, she could only make sense of material things through her immediate and spontaneous encounters with them. Her walking routine lacked any sense of purpose, or self–other interrelatedness, and hence control over its course. Instead of being *to* the world, she remained immersive, as she walked. For residents with cognitive impairments, the facets of deliberately observing and describing cease to emerge in the process of walking. They have become lost. Life is, in effect, a matter of being-*in*-the-world for Mrs Sage.

The haphazard walking of Mrs Sage was regarded by staff as maladaptive and dysfunctional because she could no longer relate to material things and persons around her or walk safely in an organized fashion. Yet, Mrs Sage was still able to walk, continuously, and on her own. This leads us to think, then, that despite her cognitive impairments, Mrs Sage could still be 'in touch', sensuously if not cognitively, with her surroundings, through her persistent walking habit. Returning to Ingold's idea that moving, observing and describing are parallel facets of the same process of walking, we might conclude that, for Mrs Sage and residents like her, instead of being alive *to* the world, they are being alive *in* the world – *in*corporated and *in*tegrated into the lifeworlds of the nursing home environment – without the capabilities of reflective observation and description.

Walking while being immersive may also involve a dimension of being observant, not reflectively but affectively. In his Preface to the 2022 edition of *Being Alive*, Ingold revisits his notion of being observant to the world. He writes:

> To observe a stone does not mean treating it as an object. Objectification, indeed, is the very opposite of observation. For what the former casts aside, the latter brings to attention. Strictly speaking, to observe is to *follow* ... through an affective coupling of the movement of one's perception with the movement of that to which it attends. This is what it means to watch, to listen and to feel. (Ingold 2022: xiii)

In this sense, in the observant eyes of Mrs Sage, a handrail or a lounge chair 'is no longer cast in the embodied form of an object in a material world. It is rather a moment in the elemental unfolding of a world of materials' (Ingold 2022: xiii).

Contrary to the biomedical conceptualization of 'wandering' as pathological and hence problematic, there is a strong argument that the seemingly aimless walking of people with dementia actually has an adaptive dimension. It keeps alive motor-sensorial-affective processes, which are fundamental to being-in-the-world, especially when a wide range of other cognitive abilities have been lost.

## At Home by Wandering

How, through her walking, could Mrs Sage feel at home in the nursing home? To answer this question, I will now turn to how Mrs Sage walks. Mrs Sage neither walked nor ran in the usual fashion. Instead of making contact with the floor from heel to toe and swinging her legs alternately, she touched the floor with only the front part of her soles and propelled herself forwards with very short intervals between strides. It was not an easy task for carers to assist Mrs Sage because as soon as her feet touched the floor, she would take off like a sudden gust of wind. The carers had to run to catch up with her. The difficulty of chasing after Mrs Sage was not just on account of her speed; it was more to do with the unusual rhythm of her gait, which gave carers problems when trying to walk along with her. For healthy able-bodied adults, the movements involved in walking are usually symmetrical: step length, cadence, torso movement, and ankle, knee, hip and pelvis motion are equal on the right and left sides, which gives a rhythmic walking pattern. But Mrs Sage lurched from side to side in uneven strides: one long, one short, one short, one long, then short again. The loss of symmetry in motion and timing between left and right sides was a sign of the breakdown of motor control of her gait, due to neurological or musculoskeletal damage.

Mrs Sage walked fast, leaning forward without seeming to bend her knees, which made her gait jerky and unsteady. To compound the leaning forward posture, there was also a side-to-side swing of her body as she moved. She swung towards the left when her left leg was off the floor pointing forward. She swung to the right when her right leg made the same movement. The combination of the side-to-side swing and the leaning forward movement made her walking so unstable that anyone watching would be in constant fear that she might have a fall at any minute.

But amazingly, Mrs Sage had fewer falls than one might expect. She seemed to intuitively adapt and maintain her strange bipedal gait despite her damaged bodily coordination. Her small strides were what made it possible for her to swap her supporting leg from left to right, and vice versa, thus stopping her from over-swinging to either side, which might have led to a fall. In this process, Mrs Sage navigated her way around using the material things available to her, knowing them preconsciously as they aided her walking. I noticed that she stopped her lurching forward movement adroitly, using objects within reach, such as the handrails in the corridors or the sofas in the lounge area. She did not look for the handrails; she stretched her left arm to her left to feel for the handrail when she walked down the left side of the corridor. When she walked down the right side, she reached out to her right. Her whole body, not just her arms, would seem to crunch onto the handrail as soon as it was in her grip. She did not respond to staff requests to 'sit down on this chair'. She sat herself onto a sofa or lounge chair when she happened to pass one. Then she would throw herself into the lounge chair and fit her body into the shape of the chair at the moment it embraced her. Throughout the day, Mrs Sage walked constantly along the corridors, occasionally sitting herself into chairs or clinging on to handrails to catch her breath. The corridors, the handrails and the chairs became ready to support her feet, hands and body, simply whenever they were encountered. Her engagement with convenient objects did not involve explicit awareness of their properties. With no conscious thought or planning, Mrs Sage seemed to fit into an alternative network of purposes, functions, fluid relations and perpetual movements.

In a coordinated natural flow, all Mrs Sage's bodily movements, including those involved in walking, are operating in the dimension of instrumental attention or 'subsidiary awareness', to use Polanyi's term (1958: vii, 91). This leads her to be able to 'feel' what is around her through the positions and movements of her body parts. Merging the matrix of sensory properties of place with her 'feeling awareness' of the exterior world, Mrs Sage was kept alive in a web of connectedness. In and through walking, Mrs Sage weaved herself into the lived fabric of the nursing home environment.

Living in a care facility provided Mrs Sage with a safe environment and organized assistance. Her excessive random walking was only made safe in a controlled 'wanderer-friendly' environment – created from the material things (handrails and chairs) and the collective efforts of carers, other residents and visitors, which meshed into an assemblage of care. Without staff paying close attention to the objects and persons in her path, Mrs Sage would surely have lost control of her movements. While severe cognitive impairments rendered her walking non-purposive, it was precisely by virtue of the excessiveness and repetitiveness that she was able to sensorially incorporate and become at home with her surroundings.

## Beyond Wandering

Seeking an understanding of the so-called problematic behaviours of residents with dementia, Algase and colleagues suggest that 'wandering' is in effect 'the need-driven, dementia-compromised behaviours which may express or embody the cognitively impaired person's goal or needs' (1996: 11). Considering wandering as an expression of a need, just like ordinary walking, the authors suggest that residents who wander need either to achieve a goal or to respond to the sensory stimuli in their environments.

They wander because their ways of achieving a goal or responding to a stimulus are compromised due to their cognitive impairments.

As I have discussed, a goal can be understood within the person–world relational framework as an object constructed apart from self, yet with which one wishes to form a connection. The word 'need' is often used to describe the experience of people wanting a change of their relationships with what they wish for; for example, from afar to proximate. German philosopher Hans Jonas suggests that both perception and desire put the living being in touch with what is spatially and temporally far away: 'The spatial breach between subject and object, which is provisionally crossed by perception, is at the same time the temporal breach between need and satisfaction, which is provisionally crossed by emotion (desire) and is practically filled in by movement' (2003: 206 as in Barbaras 2008: 10). Here, Jonas uses the word 'desire' to describe what is consciously experienced as a desire *for* something: a psychological event when one feels motivated to move towards an object.

For residents with cognitive competence, like Mrs Casey, what she wants could be described as a goal with a name, or an image, such as a dining area. Her walking to the dining area can be considered, recollected, anticipated, scheduled and implemented through the mental construct of a goal. As analysed earlier using Ingold's (2011) notion of ordinary walking as moving, observing and describing, in relation to Mrs Casey, the spatial gap between herself and her goal is compensated for by her mental activity.

Similarly, Algase and colleagues (1996) think that residents like Mrs Sage are driven by a goal or a need. They suggest that even wandering is needs-driven, and that residents with dementia are also motivated, either by a goal in the rational sense or as a response to sensory stimuli in their immediate environments in a physiological sense. But precisely how residents with dementia are able to do this is somewhat of a mystery. From my own observations, I find the idea of 'wandering' as a 'need-driven behaviour' simplistic and reductive as a way of describing the walking of people with dementia.

According to the authors above, wandering can be a response to something in a person's immediate environment, such as a sudden noise or bright light, or a shrinking response to a feeling of being crowded. The term 'response' could be looked at in two ways. First, it may be thought of as brief and episodic, with a clear beginning and end. Once the need to approach or withdraw is satisfied, the person stops moving. Second, it may be thought of as an immediate encounter of sensory incorporation. In responding to others, one does not have time to form thoughts about them. Connection comes through movements of the body. Another material thing or being cannot be represented as a goal in such fleeting encounters. One can hardly tell what the other *is* in passing.

Returning to the example of Mrs Sage, we saw that her walking was continuous, without clear indications of movements towards a goal or, indeed, prolonged responsive movement to sensory stimuli. I noticed that Mrs Sage, and other residents with dementia who wandered, did exhibit some approaching or repelling movements; for example, approaching a gathering of residents having high tea, or shrinking away from a male resident who appeared aggressive. Yet rather than representing a collection of separate, disparate episodes, the approaching or repelling movements appeared to be part of her ongoing process of walking among others through environment. In her habit of walking, Mrs Sage and material things or beings encountered one another continuously, as connected syntheses. Seen in the light of Deleuze and Guattari's conceptual framework of desiring-production (1977), this kind of walking should not be understood as responding but rather, as suggested by Ingold (2017), as *corresponding*. This explains how material things – a handrail and a pair of hands – are acting as productive machines, coupled and drawn into a single tangible entity. Holding a handrail may be felt by an ordinary person as a seeking of safety; but for those affected by dementia, like Mrs Sage, the intense flow of stimuli she experiences may lead her to be attracted towards another opening, before she can create the 'thingness' of a handrail in the mind. The walking of Mrs Sage did not involve any of the usual facets of observing, thinking and describing. So it was neither constructed goals nor sensory stimuli that led to her non-stop walking. Neither was it need-driven, because she was unable to perceive a particular need or comprehend what was meant by meeting a need. If Mrs Sage had a 'need' for walking, it must have been unspecific and unsatisfiable. Her manner of walking was rhizomatic. It had no predefined starting or ending point, no predetermined centre, no pre-structured system, but rather, it suggested new 'potentialities of becoming' (Deleuze and Guattari 1988: 290). How Mrs Sage walked reflected the immanent possibilities and potentialities for actualizing the very nature of human mobility and, more importantly, for revealing the invisible relations between people, materials and their surroundings.

For staff working in an aged care facility, how to get from A to B is a matter of task, time and efficiency. Course, timing and frequency are an essential part of their work. They come and go in a straight line, pushing a wheelchair, a lifter or a medication trolley. Aimless walking is thought to be something to do with getting lost. For many of the staff, walking is mostly a means of travelling over a certain distance and that is all. In light of their assumption that walking is only a means of self-transportation, carers will view the walking of residents with dementia in a way that is stereotyped and oversimplified, since it applies the neuropathological interpretative model, which, as we have discussed, refers to walking as wandering, and it is seen as a common symptom of dementia.

Nevertheless, as Janelle Taylor suggests in her autoethnography, people affected by Alzheimer's, like her own mother, have their 'own experience of the world that is different from' that of people around them, and that experience is 'interesting in its own way' (2008: 327). To illustrate, she draws on the account of Morris Friedell, who is himself affected by Alzheimer's, describing how: 'I find myself more visually sensitive ... Everything seems richer: lines, planes, contrast. It is a wonderful compensation. ... We [who have Alzheimer's disease] can appreciate clouds, leaves, flowers as we never did before' (Shenk 2001: 193 as in Taylor 2008: 327).

Through her experience of walking slowly with her mother, hand in hand, around the neighbourhood of the facility where her mother lives, Taylor comes to realize that while 'the loosening of memory' may leave her mother 'stranded in the present moment', it 'also allows her to inhabit it more fully' (2008: 372). They may have no cognitive impairment but are too caught up in the rush of their everyday lives. In the case of Mrs Sage, she could inhabit the nursing home environment by walking, and this was more than simply getting from one place to another. For nursing home residents with dementia, the act of walking should never be reduced to a symptom of brain pathology. Instead, in and through walking, they could discover and re-create a sense of home.

# 3 WALKING OUT OF THE FREEZE

## The Frozen Gait of Mr Harris

The vignette in the Introduction describes how Mr Harris, a man with Parkinson's disease, could feel just right in and through walking, able to become at home in the nursing home despite the constraints of living in a secure care facility. In this chapter, I want to examine how his walking changed over time as his mind and body declined. Mr Harris is one of the few residents with whom I formed a bond in the initial stage of my fieldwork. I met him when we were both negotiating the 'roundabout' at the intersection of three adjoining wings of residents' rooms (see Figure 3.1).

A stranger to the facility, neither resident nor staff, I felt self-conscious and out of place as I paced back and forth there. People gave me inquisitive looks as they walked by. No one stopped to talk to me. I felt awkward and lost. Then Mr Harris arrived on the scene. With the aid of a red 4-wheeled walker, he walked cautiously, leaning forward, with his neck bent so that his head slightly drooped over his chest. Stopping in front of me, only two steps away, he inspected my badge and asked: 'What are you doing in *this* place?' There was a sense of authority in his voice, which was slow, deep, yet strangely flat. He wore a solemn expression that made his face look mask-like. 'I'm a student learning about aged care'. I kept my answer short and simple. 'Do you want to get a job here when you finish?' he asked. 'I am still learning. I'm not sure whether I will work here,' I told him. 'It's not an easy job working here,' he said, sombrely. I nodded in agreement.

He slowly turned his walker towards the corridor, as if about to leave. Before he walked off, he patted the handlebar of his walker, using his right palm and said, 'You have your job to do; I have mine.' As my fieldwork continued, I realized what Mr Harris meant by referring to walking as his job. Often left by staff to meander on his own, he would observe people coming and going, and he would regularly reach out and engage with them.

Walking extended Mr Harris' social world beyond the parameters of his room, and it was how he occupied himself in the nursing home. When his bodily condition allowed, he wanted to spend time on his feet. In the

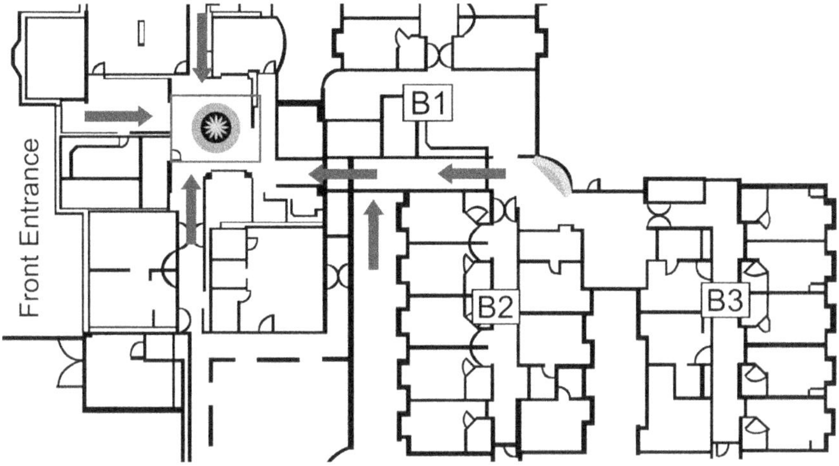


FIGURE 3.1. The 'roundabout' on the ground floor. The circle with a grey star in a black circle marks the seat in the middle of the roundabout; the square surrounding the circles marks the roundabout area; the arrows show people's walking routes towards the roundabout. Illustration: Michael Tianze Zhang. Published with permission.

early days of my fieldwork, I seldom saw him sitting, except for a cup of tea, a meal or a break: he used to walk so much that staff no longer paid attention to his presence, as long as they thought he could walk safely on his own.

In the lifeworld of Mr Harris, walking around while checking on people was an occupation. This notion of walking as a commitment that is centrally placed in residents' lives resonates with the accounts of T.D., a North American nursing home resident. In a conversation with the ethnographer, T.D. asserted that residents '… could help themselves and be happy' in the nursing home if they could 'get walking' (Vesperi 2003: 88). For nursing home residents like Mr Harris and T.D., walking is productive and adds meaning. It is more than simply passing time or wandering. But with their physical deterioration, walking, as nursing home residents frequently expressed through their words and gestures, could require a great deal of effort and assistance.

As the two previous chapters demonstrated, for nursing home residents with bodily impairments, the act of walking can never be taken for granted. Becoming mobile takes time and care. Halfway into my fieldwork, Mr Harris started having increasing difficulties with walking, and in walking alongside him, I noticed that he was gradually slowing down, and his stride was shortening. Sometimes he began to shuffle – dragging his feet along the carpet to a standstill – before he started walking again. He could

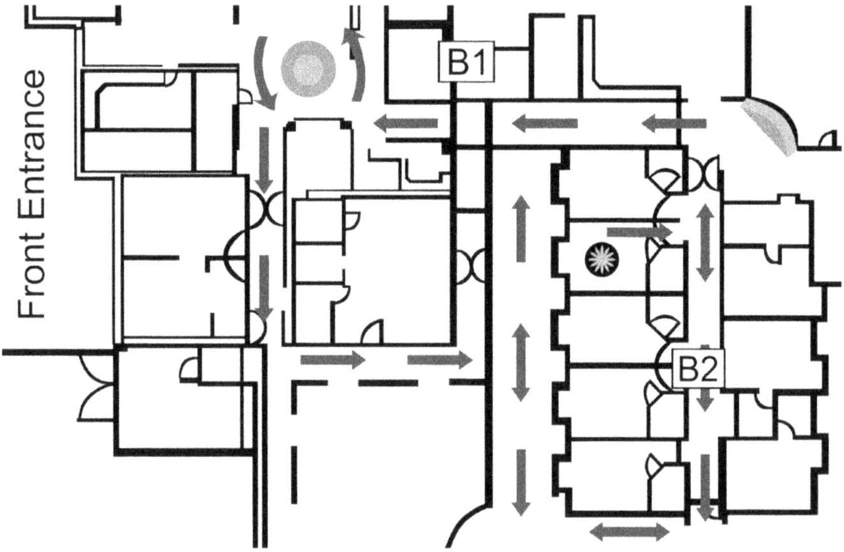


FIGURE 3.2. Mr Harris' daily walking routine. The circle marks the seat in the middle of the roundabout; the grey star in a black circle marks Mr Harris' room; the arrows show Mr Harris' daily walking routes. Illustration: Michael Tianze Zhang. Published with permission.

usually walk for a few metres in a string of even strides. Then, as soon as he looked down at his own feet, he started shuffling in small steps, as if the sight of his feet moving interfered with their movement.

His walking deteriorated rapidly as his Parkinson's disease further developed. He constantly struggled with initiating first steps: unable to move his feet forward even with some visible effort from his lower limbs exerting force. It was as if his feet were glued to the floor or were too heavy to lift and move forward as he wished. Even on occasions when he could slightly lever his feet from the floor, he could barely shift his weight from one foot to the other to create a forward movement. Like a stutterer who has difficulty generating fluent utterances, who pauses before speaking or repeats the first part of a word several times, he had difficulty generating coherent movements. In the nursing home, staff referred to Mr Harris' unusual form of walking as 'the frozen gait', a symptom associated with Parkinson's disease.

Mr Harris struggled to produce the concerted movements necessary for walking. On some occasions, an increased forward lean meant he walked with a progressive quickening of steps, which might have led him to fall forward, if not assisted by staff to slow down. He regularly had the frozen gait episodes when he attempted to walk. Sometimes he also froze on the spot and came to a sudden halt. This happened when a particular thing in the environment came closer to him as he walked towards it, such as stepping through a doorway, attempting to turn a corner or approaching a chair. The freezing lasted for a few seconds or as long as several minutes. Once his attention shifted from the object in his path, his walking resumed. Although the sudden halt was usually fleeting, his walking was losing its natural rhythm and flow, meaning he was increasingly unstable and at risk of falling.

As his Parkinson's disease progressed, it was as if Mr Harris and his ability to walk became switched off. As I will later describe in more detail, this was also how clinical staff conceptualized his loss of movement. Observing how residents lose their capacity to move led me to wonder what had happened to the inner drive that had previously instigated them to get up and dressed and do their 'job'; in Mr Harris's case, that meant patrolling the corridors of the nursing home. In the following section, I use Deleuze and Guattari's (1977, 1988) notion of desire as a productive lens to examine the tensions between walking and not walking. In doing so, I consider how, despite being seemingly switched off from walking, Mr Harris was entwined in an assemblage of care that propelled him to keep moving and walking.

## Parkinson's Disease: Living in Tension between Walking and Not Walking

Mr Harris was admitted into the aged care facility due to the progression of his Parkinson's disease. He was known to his family and friends as a 'good mate': intelligent, energetic, cheerful and easy-going. Yet, in the eyes of staff, he transformed into a stern, sullen and stubborn resident with whom they felt it was difficult to relate. It may be that their feelings about Mr Harris arose not merely due to his personality changes but because of the impression given from the flat tone of his voice and facial masking, both of which are symptoms of Parkinson's disease. His face showed little expression because his facial muscles had become immobilized. Mr Harris was even losing his ability to perform automatic movements, such as blinking and smiling, and consequently he always appeared uninterested and bored. However, as described above, Mr Harris had once been very interested in engaging with other people.

The progression of his Parkinson's disease also transformed the appearance of Mr Harris in other ways. He had had a long career in the construction industry as an electrical engineer and was an enthusiastic participant in many sports, including cricket, football and running. Posed with fellow athletes, in the fading photographs displayed in his room, you could see that Mr Harris was once a tall man with an erect and powerful build. Now he looked much shorter with his forward-flexed posture, head pointing forward and arms hanging down in front. Forward-flexed posture is caused by weakened lower muscles of the back. Damage to the brain can inhibit proper flexion and extension in the muscles necessary for maintaining an upright posture. Upon admission, Mr Harris was assessed for mobility and prescribed a 4-wheeled walker to assist with his walking and protect against falls. Like Mrs Casey, Mr Harris discovered that the walker was a good fit for him. The support of the walker compensated for his forward-leaning tendency and stopped him from falling forwards.

After frequent occurrences of 'the freeze', Mr Harris was stopped from walking on his own without assistance from staff. He then spent most of his days sitting in a lounge chair snoozing. When sleeping, Mr Harris could not lie back in a semi-recumbent position on the couch, as many other residents do. His Parkinsonism was making his posture more and more rigid. His arms were as stiff as dry sticks and his muscles as hard as rocks. Sitting stiffly, with legs crossed and arms folded for long periods, emphasized his frozen statue-like appearance.

He also experienced involuntary movements of his fingers, or 'rest tremor'. The shaking of his right-side fingers was most apparent when Mr Harris sat still watching television. Unable to consciously exert control over his movements in forms of initiation or inhibition – people with Parkinson's disease lose control over their muscle movements – distal extremities appear to move of their own accord, as if expressing some innermost urge of the person to reach out.

Ordinarily, in inhibiting unintended movements in a standing posture, the whole body is involved in a conflation of bodily processes that keep the muscles relaxed while maintaining an upright posture. This requires as much if not more active and accurate control as producing the movements themselves. In the case of Mr Harris, stiffness of his limbs was caused by increased muscle tone. This is the result of excessive and continuous contraction of muscles, which actually reflects preparation of the muscles for activity but fails to actualize into the act of walking. In regard to Mr Harris's hand tremor, we might hypothesize that while the brain's control over the physiology of movement was largely blocked, the intensity of neurological flow found its release at the distal extremities of hands.

The existence of a deeply embodied innermost drive to move is obviously demonstrated in residents' persistent attempts to stand up and take steps. When Mr Harris was awake and sitting on a wingback lounge chair, he used to move his buttocks to the edge of the chair and push himself up, as if he was trying to rise to tear himself away from the embracing comfort of the chair. Occasionally, he could stand up and take a few steps, with support from something close by, such as the small all-purpose wheelie table. Yet, his risk of falling increased on such occasions because in moving away from the lounge chair, he might have ended up making a hard landing on the floor. The repetitive attempts of residents to change their position from sitting to standing, or vice versa, is conceived by staff as 'agitative behaviour'; that is, a behaviour described in gerontological literature as 'restless behaviour, or improper physical and verbal actions that may cause trouble for family members, caregivers and other service users' (Ijaopo 2017: 1). Staff explained that agitated residents 'keep trying and forget that they can no longer stand and walk on their own'. The medical discourse on agitative behaviour, or agitation, together with staff remarks, present these repetitive and persistent movements as symptoms: the manifestations of residents' declining mobility and cognition.

Parkinson's disease as a clinical entity is considered a progressive, neurodegenerative condition that results from the destruction of nerve cells in the brain area called the basal ganglia. It is hypothesized in neurological research that the basal ganglia normally exerts a constant inhibitory influence on movement control systems, preventing them from becoming active at inappropriate times, such as when moving is seen as potentially dangerous. The role that the basal ganglia plays is to reduce inhibition for the required constellations of movements, thereby releasing them for activation. The experience of voluntary movement comes from the smooth communication – using a neurotransmitter called dopamine – between the basal ganglia and other parts of the brain. When the cells that produce dopamine die, the signal to move does not get communicated and transmitted to the muscles.

Setting aside such biomedical conceptualizations, I am choosing here to consider Parkinson's disease as an interruption in ordinary everyday processes of moving. For residents with Parkinson's disease, the urge to walk does not necessarily lead to walking. The desire to move meets the opposing force of withdrawal, causing blockages in movement that limit one's capacity to walk. What is conceptualized as symptoms in Parkinson's disease – limb stiffness or slow movement (bradykinesia) – could be regarded as a lack of natural flow of movements. That lack, as Deleuze and Guattari (1977) suggest, is 'a countereffect of desire', which indicates the rise of the force of withdrawal over the productive power of desire. In voluntarily standing, the change of position from sitting to standing may or may not become actualized, depending on the moment-to-moment bodily condition, which is constantly fluctuating for those with Parkinson's disease. In approaching residents' experiences of Parkinson's from the perspective of desiring-production, the so-called symptoms can be understood as an interruption of the desiring-production processes.

The frozen gait of Mr Harris can also be understood as a particular manifestation of the desiring-production process. Purposefully walking ordinarily involves focal awareness, the conscious selection of an aim, path and time to walk, combined with subsidiary awareness, the preconscious coordination of many bodily processes: leading to the actual performance of walking. While focal awareness is at play in our purposeful walking, it is subsidiary awareness that leads to our flow of fluent movements. The experience of walking as an action of control, certainty and easiness thus comes from the integrated functioning of two levels of consciousness. However, when there is an intention to move but an absence of executed voluntary movements, this is an indication that the ordinarily concerted functioning of consciousness is disrupted. The frozen gait of Mr Harris indicated that there was a disjuncture between what was intended – namely, the initiation of walking – and the execution of movements: his actual taking of steps. The wish of Mr Harris to walk was temporarily overridden by the over-inhibition of movement, and what was displayed was the frozen gait.

While Mrs Casey and Mr Harris were both in a similar situation in that they struggled to continue walking, Mrs Casey, with her diabetes, was able to relearn walking whereas Mr Harris was losing the ability to walk on his own. His transferring of position from sitting to standing could not be easily actualized, and his attempts failed repeatedly. He often fell back into the depths of a high back lounge chair, and exhausted after his struggle, he would fall asleep again.

Consequently, sitting in one spot for prolonged periods had a significant impact on Mr Harris. Staff spoke about him as 'going downhill' and deteriorating rapidly. He became mute most of the time and unresponsive towards his carers. Increasingly, Mr Harris was seen as having sunk into a deep solitude, and he was described as having become 'part of the furniture' or a 'statue', to use the carers' words. Compared to his earlier self, who was mobile and engaging with other people around him, the now non-walking Mr Harris became isolated, withdrawn and uninterested. According to nursing staff, Mr Harris had developed the medical condition of apathy, in which residents appear to have no motivational capacities, tendencies or dispositions. The staff concluded his capacity to walk was lost due to his neurological condition of Parkinson's disease, and that prolonged sitting had greatly reduced his remaining capacities to the point that he could no longer walk. In short, Mr Harris was thought to be incapable of walking, and as staff remarked, he was totally dependent on their assistance to 'get walked'.

My own observations suggest that residents with movement disorders, like Mr Harris, may live in a kind of tension between walking and not walking. When Mr Harris became increasingly apathetic and withdrawn, did it not indicate that he was experiencing more blockages in the flow of intensity and a gradual breakdown of the syntheses in desiring-production? The next section explores how other material things, such as his medication, may have impacted his movements and, indeed, his ability to walk.

## The 'On-and-Off' Phenomenon

Taking medication plays a pivotal role in reducing the impact of Parkinson's disease. Mr Harris was prescribed two-hourly levodopa (a dopamine replacement) to reduce his stiffness, pain, tremor and other related symptoms. During a training session on care for residents living with dementia, the clinical nurse used the example of Mr Harris to show the importance of being strict with medication schedules. She explained that while Parkinson's medication might help to boost dopamine levels in the brain, it could only work for a short amount of time. For this reason, doctors usually prescribe a two-hourly schedule of medication for Parkinson's patients. Effective management of Parkinson's symptoms is dependent on getting medication on time, every time. If the two-hourly schedule is not closely followed, residents would be likely to experience the fluctuation of symptoms that is called the 'on-and-off' phenomenon.

The on-and-off phenomenon in Parkinson's disease refers to this switch between being able to move and unable to move and is related to medication dosage. The switch will often occur at the end of the dose period, when the medication is wearing off. It will result in worsening of motor function or, less commonly, will produce sudden and unpredictable motor fluctuations. When Parkinson's medication is working well, the patient's symptoms are well controlled. This is called the 'on' time. When symptoms are not well controlled, or patients do not respond to medication, this is called the 'off' time.

Mr Harris showed symptom fluctuations at times when his Parkinson's medication was skipped. He had a more noticeable tremor, worse stiffness and looked more depressed. The combined effects of tremor, rigidity and joint pain could render limb movements excruciating to Mr Harris. Forty-five minutes after taking his medication, the tremor of his hand became less obvious, and his limbs became less rigid. His whole person seemed to be more relaxed and in a better mood. This was also the scheduled time for his staff-assisted walking routine. For Annie and other personal care staff, it was critical to ensure that Mr Harris had taken his Parkinson's medication before assisting him to walk. Forty-five minutes to one hour after taking his Parkinson's medication, Mr Harris was at his best to move: he was 'switched on'.

The taking of medication followed by the switching on of his voluntary movements indicate that Mr Harris experienced what I call a kind of 'fission of mind'. Parkinson's disease disrupts the connectedness between the 'decision-making' and the 'acting' parts of the neurological system. With medication working to boost dopamine levels in the brain, coherent functioning is restored temporarily. Thinking about the effect of Parkinson's medication in terms of desiring-production, it can be seen as a biochemical enhancement leading to connective synthesis in movement production, a pivotal component of caring for patients with Parkinson's disease.

In contrast to Mrs Casey and Mrs Sage, who continued to walk mostly through their own efforts to move, Mr Harris could not walk without being 'switched on' by engagement with other material things and persons, including the chemical agents in his Parkinson's medication. If residents like Mrs Casey and Mrs Sage could feel just right in walking, mostly on their own, was it possible for Mr Harris to also feel right when he was 'walked' by carers? If so, in what ways could assisted walking (either by walking aid or staff) contribute to a sense of being right, and hence at home? For a better understanding of how Mr Harris could continue walking, I now turn to the actual process of Mr Harris's walking and describe in detail how carers assisted him to walk out of his freeze. This demonstrates how *assemblages of care* – synthesized efforts of Mr Harris and other material things and persons – could contribute to Mr Harris' continuing to walk, through the process of desiring-production.

## Out of the Freeze

When Mr Harris was assisted to walk, it was a dynamic and sensuous activity, filled with sounds, expressions and gestures as well as movements. Standing to the left of Mr Harris, Annie put her own left foot forward and said: 'Left foot first, Mr Harris. One step forward.' Mr Harris copied Annie's foot movement by moving his left foot forward. 'Well done, Mr Harris,' Annie said. She then put her right foot forward for Mr Harris to copy that movement. After the first three to four steps of slow and awkward imitation, Mr Harris started walking more naturally. Walking together, Annie started humming the nursery rhyme 'Mary had a little lamb'. Stepping to the beat of the song, Mr Harris was now walking smoothly, but when they approached the lounge area, Mr Harris suddenly froze and came to a halt. At this location, the colour of the carpet changed from a dark pattern to a brighter flowery design and the change seemed to faze him. Putting her own foot horizontally in front of Mr Harris, Annie told him 'Step onto my foot.' With some hesitation, Mr Harris did so. Annie then stood in front of Mr Harris and walked backwards, saying, 'Look at me, Mr Harris', and 'Left, right, left, right' to keep his attention on moving. She then led Mr Harris across the threshold and into the lounge area. She had helped him to literally walk out of his freeze.

I observed closely how Mr Harris became distracted as soon as he looked down at his own feet: he started shuffling in small steps as if seeing his own feet had interfered with their movements. As discussed in Chapter 1, using Polanyi's (1958) concepts of subsidiary and focal awareness, the coordination of the constellations of bodily movements involved in walking relies on the seamless flow of operational consciousness across preconscious and conscious levels. In ordinary walking, one's feet and their movements are usually out of the person's view and merge into the operation of subsidiary awareness. When we look at our own feet, the feet and their movements are isolated and scrutinized at another level, that of focal awareness. In the case of Mrs Casey, perceptually monitoring the continuous movements of her feet using focal awareness played a pivotal role in her careful walking. The involvement of focal awareness in the walking of Mrs Casey was essential because to walk safely the interrupted operation of subsidiary awareness needs to be compensated for with conscious attention. In having control over the initiation, continuation and termination of her walking, Mrs Casey could feel just right and continue her safe walking. In the process of her walking, both her physical impairments and cognitive competence were affecting how she walked and how she felt about her walking. Her diabetic feet motivated Mrs Casey to create a careful way of walking.

Conversely, in the case of Mr Harris, the sight of his own feet moving created a rupture in the connective syntheses, which interrupted his walking. To draw his attention away from his own feet and start a new flow following the ruptured movement, Mr Harris needed assistance from Annie. By walking backwards in front of him and counting rhythmically, Annie helped Mr Harris to move his gaze away from his feet. As soon as he looked up at Annie, he resumed walking. As shown through the examples of Mrs Casey and Mr Harris, bodily impairments can be seen as blockages leading to ruptures in rhizomatic becomings of their movements. Yet, as shown in how Annie assisted Mr Harris to resume walking, a rupture is never the ending point of a rhizome. As Deleuze and Guattari (1988) suggest, new pathways often appear in response to ruptures, which renders bodily impairments a force that is both constitutive and differentiating.

Precisely how Mr Harris and carers walked together is intriguing. Although he was slow, shuffling and frozen from time to time, with the support of his wheelie walker and in the company of Annie, Mr Harris could walk to her rhythmical counting for a short distance in a string of even strides. Mr Harris' movements were affected by the presence and movements of Annie. She used humming and counting; she shifted his attention from moving his legs forward to stepping onto a given target – her own foot on the floor. That combination of her counting and placing her own foot in front of him had enabled Mr Harris, both in a temporal and spatial sense, to step forward, following her footsteps.

The walking of Mr Harris and that of Annie were intertwined in multisensory processes as they moved in relation to each other. The sight of his own feet, or of the little gap between the carpet and the timber floor, ceased to form a disjuncture that would freeze Mr Harris's movements. Instead, the voice of Annie, the presence of her foot, the momentum and the velocity of his walker merged into connective syntheses. While Mr Harris cared about continuing to walk, Annie cared for him to feel just right in and through walking. Routinely walking together is an activity that involves connectedness with other people. It also engenders a sense of belonging, which is at the core of feeling at home.

Mr Harris may not have understood those deeper implications of a staff-assisted walking routine, which is institutionally offered as a usual practice of mobility care. But that sense of connection led him to move and, by extension, feel at home. Annie's able body became a supportive extension of his arms and legs as he followed her instructions. Her unspoken message was: 'Go on walking, this place is safe to move through.' The cause of freezing in Parkinson's patients is comparable to defensive freezing in life-threatening situations, when a sense of threat and uncertainty, felt in the body, leads to fear and despair (Roelofs 2017). In such a situation, the multisensory presence and engagement of a friendly other person acts like a shelter from some unknown and terrible danger. Mr Harris thus was thawed and able to walk out of the spell of inhibition, avoidance and isolation imposed by his Parkinson's disease.

## Staff-Assisted Walking: Routines and Ruptures

As we think about how Mr Harris was able to walk, assisted by carers, it becomes clear that the efforts, sensations and movements of Mr Harris and his carers were intertwined. For residents like Mr Harris, staff participation is a crucial element in their 'becoming-walking'. As his frozen gait was thawed and freed up, Mr Harris's whole-body syntheses reignited. Once again he could find his footing and, through that, regain a sense of home through affectively and sensorially relating to another human being.

Other material things and persons may also have facilitated the process; for example, his use of medication. Clearly, the two-hourly dosage of his Parkinson's medication also played a pivotal role in Mr Harris's walking routine and was another essential element in his overall care.

As illustrated by this account of Mr Harris' assisted walking, there was no one factor or intervention – be it a walking routine, a medication regime or assistance by a carer – that could enable residents with movement disorders, like Mr Harris, to continue to walk. It took an assemblage of care – the involvement of many material things and persons – to walk Mr Harris out of his freeze. The efforts of Mr Harris himself can be seen as a type of self-care: taking his medication, following staff instructions and making each and every step forward. The example of Mr Harris clearly shows that a staff-assisted walking routine can be a beneficial process, where an innermost drive to move, supported by other material things in an assemblage of care, can enable residents to walk.

The staff-assisted walking routine worked well to assist Mr Harris with his walking; however, it had some limitations. As a key component of mobility care, staff-assisted walking is classed as a service item provided to residents, and a task assigned to staff, to be carried out at a fixed time – for example, before or after lunch – for a fixed duration of 10 to 15 minutes. So Mr Harris was only assisted to walk for 10 to 15 minutes a day. 'That's all we have time to do,' staff claimed. Instead of walking when he felt the urge to move, Mr Harris only walked as scheduled. While staff commented that a staff-assisted walking routine 'works' in that it assisted Mr Harris to walk safely, they also admitted that its use was limited by the time they could allocate. So, in effect, Mr Harris was for most of the time not walking. This deepens our understanding of the staff-assisted walking routine. While such a routine can be useful in assisting residents to walk safely, it is not, as staff pointed out, able to assist residents to walk *whenever they would like to.* While a staff-assisted walking routine works well as part of an important assemblage of care, the term 'routine' shows that its usefulness is limited by the facility's overarching prescheduled temporal structure.

This understanding is important for residents with immobilizing conditions, like Mr Harris, because a deeper understanding of their experiences of staff-assisted walking routines is crucial for service providers in terms of care allocation and prioritization. In the following chapter, I extend this discussion on the staff-assisted walking routine to examine the multiple versions of care in nursing homes.

# 4 LIVING IN THE TENSION BETWEEN WALKING AND NOT WALKING

## Unable to Walk

When residents approach the end of their lives, continuing to walk often becomes a struggle. No longer able to walk safely on their own or stand up and balance on their feet, they spend most of the day sitting in chairs. Mr Dixon was one such resident. Every time I saw Mr Dixon, he was sitting down alone in his room. Given its proximity to the central communal area, and with the door wide open during the day, people could catch a glimpse of him from the corridor as they passed by. Sitting in front of the window in a 'comfort chair' specifically designated for residents who sit for long hours, Mr Dixon was often asleep. Framed by the curtains of his window, he looked like an artwork in a gallery – with his head drooping onto his chest, his arms folded and legs crossed – he remained sitting in the same posture for hours. With eyebrows locked together and lips pursed, an expression of anguish seemed etched onto his deeply wrinkled face, giving him a statue-like appearance. His motionless form was in stark contrast to the world of perpetual movement going on right outside his door: people walking past, some easily, others with difficulty; some moving fast, others slowly; some who could move on their own and others who needed assistance. When asleep in his chair, Mr Dixon appeared to be insulated in a separate world from that of the people around him. Although he maintained his connections with the world by breathing in and out, and by the sense of touch that came from the pressure of body–chair contact, in this state of being 'shut down', he was largely unresponsive towards other material things and beings around him.

Mr Dixon was not alone in his habit of sleeping for long periods during the day. In the facility, residents who could no longer walk safely on their own tended to just sit. Sitting seemed to be the primary mode of daily living for many nursing home residents, especially those who suffered from debilitating health problems that impeded their movements. Although residents were regularly assisted by staff to move around while sitting in a wheelchair, to take part in meals and activities, at other times they sat in comfort chairs in their rooms or in the communal lounge. Some spent most of their time during the day sitting in front of the television watching cartoons or musicals. Like Mr Dixon, residents often fell asleep while sitting down and staying still: in fact, they slept on and off during the whole day. In sitting and sleeping, they showed little interest in what was going on around them.

My observations of what staff describe as residents 'sitting down, staying still and snoozing' are in line with research findings from other nursing home studies. In a study with 723 resident participants from seven Netherlands nursing homes, residents were usually observed to remain in lying or sitting positions (range: 89%–92%) and mainly noted to be sleeping, doing nothing or watching television (Den Ouden et al. 2015). In the first study to measure activity and sedentary patterns in aged care residents in Australia, monitored data indicates that residents are highly sedentary, spending an average 85% (>12 hours/day) of waking hours sitting or lying, with nearly half of this sedentary time spent in prolonged bouts of at least 60 minutes (Reid et al. 2013).

In contrast to residents who regularly stand up and walk, residents who sit for prolonged periods are considered by health researchers as inactive (Den Ouden et al. 2015; Reid et al. 2013). But in walking and sitting with residents, I came to see their seemingly stationary positions as far more complex and dynamic than the health research implies. This can be seen through the example of 'the ladies sitting in the communal area'. The same group of elderly women always sat together in the couches located in the communal area from morning teatime (10 AM) to late afternoon (4 PM). They seldom talked to each other but sat quietly together, watching people coming and going. From time to time, visitors complained about being 'glared at', and staff described their sitting as a 'strange behaviour'.

As this lounge is situated at a central crossing point between the adjourning areas B1, B2 and B3, a large amount of traffic, including residents, staff and visitors, move in and out of the area (see Figure 4.1). Instead of sitting within the four walls of their individual rooms, these residents sat amidst the flows of movements of staff, sounds, visitors, trolleys, the passing breeze and wafting aromas. They were watching, hearing, smelling and feeling, while being seen. They seemed to have mingled with others in their movements while remaining seated. In sitting with these female residents daily, I came to understand that their sitting was not simply a state of being immobile and inactive, and nor was it a 'strange behaviour'. There exists an innermost drive in residents to connect and to be in touch with others and the world. They were doing this by sitting.

In anthropological work, the key feature of walking – the body itself moving while moving through the world – renders walking a unique mode of being-in-the-world. Unlike walking, both standing and sitting are at rest

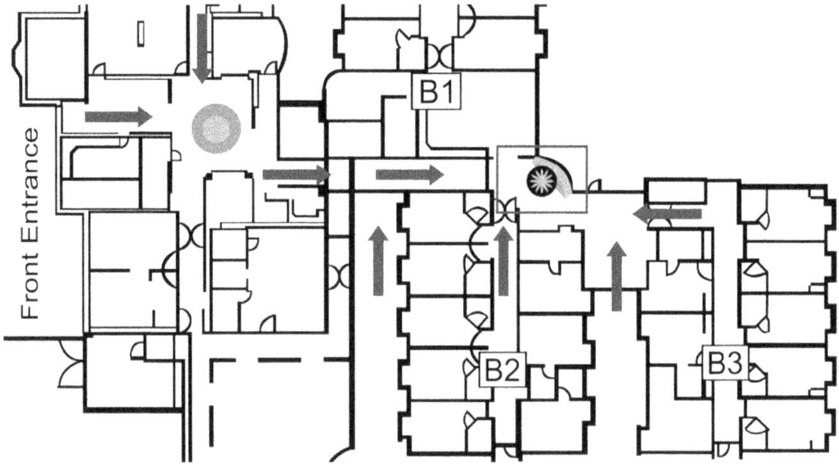


FIGURE 4.1. Location of the lounge area and people's movements around it. The semi-circle with a grey star in a black circle marks the couches in the lounge area; the rectangle around it marks the lounge area; the arrows show people's movements around the lounge area. Illustration: Michael Tianze Zhang. Published with permission.

in relation to the surroundings because no change of location is involved. Standing and sitting are positions, staying in one spot without moving away. Sitting is experienced as more sedentary than standing because what is crucial in standing – balance on one's own feet while maintaining an upright posture – is non-essential in sitting. Balancing on one's feet is not just about maintaining an upright posture. It is a matter of knowing one's position in relation to the world. Also absent from sitting is the sense of being grounded: experiencing the body as a whole from the feet up. With or without one's feet touching the ground, in sitting, one is either partially grounded or completely ungrounded.

More importantly, as this section on walking illustrates, residents' own efforts were central and indispensable in creating a right assemblage of care in the process of becoming-walking. In continuing to walk, residents could feel right and at home, being active, connected and in control. In sitting, residents seemed to have experienced the opposite: they made no effort and appeared to be inactive, disconnected and withdrawn, despite their efforts to remain connected with other people by sitting together in a communal area. If being alive, as Ingold (2011) suggests, is to move through the world, the pathway seems to arrive at a dead end when nursing home residents can no longer walk around and they are subtly encouraged to be sedentary by staff attitudes and the use of incentives to remain sitting.

When walking becomes compromised, what happens to the lives of nursing home residents, and how might their shifting states of bodily decline articulate with other persons and things to produce (or inhibit) new ways of walking and becoming at ease and at home? Is it still possible for residents who are unable to walk on their own to have a sense of being-at-home in the nursing home? Shifting our focus from the study of walking to movements involved in sitting and attempted standing, this chapter explores how limits to walking can be reconfigured through a right assemblage of care. Before so doing, I want in the next section to look at the experiences of sitting and moving in the context of certain residents with cognitive impairments due to later stages of dementia.

## Sitting Up to Move

Outside of nursing homes, 'transfer' is not an everyday word for describing movement, but in nursing homes it is often used to refer to changing a resident's physical position. Moving from one position to another is a taken-for-granted aspect of daily life among able-bodied persons. But in nursing homes, transfer, like walking, involves the whole-body movements essential to changing position, such as from sitting to standing. Rising from a chair is perhaps one of the toughest tasks. It involves moving from a static, seated position through an unstable transition phase, to a 'quasi-static' (standing) position. Successful transition requires significant motor control, momentum and coordination.

Den Ouden and colleagues' (2015) Netherlands nursing home study noted that transfers, in which the resident changes position, were rarely observed. In their study, they observed multiple positions of residents, including lying, sitting, standing, walking and transferring, at random times between 7 AM to 11 PM. Out of the total number of positions observed, only 1% related to the process of transferring from one position to another. Low incidence of transfer may indicate that residents are unable to get out of a chair on their own due to impairments. This was identified as a problem in that research because it suggests strongly that residents sitting for prolonged periods experience a high level of inactivity (Den Ouden et al. 2015: 963). In health research, sitting is considered a mode of inactivity and transfer as an activity. Den Ouden's research therefore recommends integrating physical activities of sit–stand, standing and walking into the residents' daily routine as a form of care, so that their need for activity can be met.

However, sitting is far more complex than merely staying still and inactive. Residents experience sitting in many different ways. They may remain seated during a period without a change of position; however, they will not be completely motionless unless they fall asleep. And even then, they may snore, twitch or speak. While falling asleep will clearly make them inactive, if awake, they will constantly move about in their chairs, even if they cannot make a complete transfer and rise to standing.

Unlike walking, during which one travels in distance, in making a transfer, one remains in the same spot while the body itself moves. In either making a complete transfer from sitting to standing or an incomplete transfer from sitting (attempting to stand then returning to sit), movement of the whole body is involved. As sitting is a central yet overlooked bodily practice in the lives of nursing home residents, I would like in this section to describe the nuances of sitting and its entanglement with other people and things, taking the everyday life of Mr Dixon as my example.

When Mr Dixon fell asleep while seated in his chair, he needed very little staff attention and assistance. Staff referred to these days as his 'good days'. Mr Dixon often slept during the day, mostly because he was exhausted from being hyperactive during the previous night. At night, he acted out his violent dreams, kicking, punching and shouting at the top of his voice as if he were fighting for his life. Staff described these as the 'bad nights', and they impacted on staff and other residents living in the same wing as Mr Dixon. Mr Dixon had a sleeping problem known in the field as rapid eye movement sleep behaviour disorder, which was understood as a symptom of the neurodegenerative condition of dementia with Lewy bodies. In response to action-filled dreams, such as being chased or defending himself from an attack, he threw slippers at shadows on the walls; he jumped out of bed and fought staff when they tried to bring him back into bed. He could also become severely disoriented and delusional at night. On one occasion, he wandered into another resident's room across the corridor searching for the toilet and was shocked to see a female resident lying in her bed. 'Who is that woman sleeping in my house?' he asked when the night shift carer heard the scream of the old woman and came to help.

Sometimes he hurt himself by bumping into furniture or having falls. However, worse than the bad nights, were the bad days, when he was in motion, awake and alert. Moving his buttocks to the edge of the chair and pushing down on the armrests, he constantly tried to rise from the chair, but he was usually incapable of doing transfers without help. His attempts to stand up and walk were usually unsuccessful: most of the time, he simply fell back into his chair. Yet, with obvious determination, he continued with his efforts to move.

Mr Dixon experienced two contrasting alternate modalities of sitting. First, sitting down, he would be still and drowsy. Second, if he was attempting to stand up, he would be attentive and active. From minute to minute and day to day, staff never knew for sure how well he might be able to stand up or walk. Some days he could walk with little staff assistance, knew who everyone was and would chat with his visiting families and friends. The next day he would sit for hours, as described in the vignette in the opening section, in a somnolent state, as if in a coma.

While not as extreme as Mr Dixon, I observed that many residents had intermittent phases of 'sitting down asleep' and 'sitting up to move' during any lengthy period of sitting down. With Mr Dixon, however, the incomplete transfers played a critical role in constituting his two modalities of sitting. The movement and activity that was absent when sitting returned when he sat up and tried to stand. Thus, Mr Dixon, in his later stages of dementia, was not, contrary to dominant aged care discourse, fixed in a homogeneous mode of immobility and inactivity. His shifts between sleeping and waking, or sitting down and preparing to stand, were, in the words of aged care clinicians, 'low in arousal' and 'high in activity'; they reflected an ever-changing body–world relationship. Sitting can actually represent a flow of changing positions, leading to sleep, or movement with the intention to stand up and walk. In short, for nursing home residents in the later stages of dementia, sitting is indeed a primary mode of daily living, but it is never a mode that is completely stationary.

As the descriptions of how residents experience sitting demonstrate, sitting should not be seen as a sign they have reached the limits of their ability to make movements. Rather, it needs to be understood as residents experiencing tension between the opposing forces that are constitutive to their moving or not moving. In the waking hours of Mr Dixon, he was simultaneously motivated by a drive to move and demotivated by his impaired balance, which restricted him from leaving his chair.

Mr Dixon lived this tension between moving and not moving whilst being affected by constant fluctuations of conscious awareness, cognition and movement due to dementia. This chapter demonstrates how limited mobility should not be treated as inactivity but rather as difficulties with walking. In the next section, I illustrate the 'roller coaster' of ups and downs that shaped Mr Dixon's everyday life in the nursing home before then detailing how specific arrangements of care ameliorated or amplified these tensions and assisted him to move.

## Living the 'Roller Coaster': Shifting Potentialities of Moving

In the field, residents in the later stages of dementia, like Mr Dixon, sit for long hours but are not always completely still. Their experiences of sitting are complex due to their various bodily conditions. Mr Dixon had a diagnosis of dementia with Lewy bodies before his entry into the care facility. Dementia with Lewy bodies is considered the second most prevalent cause of degenerative dementia in older people: only Alzheimer's disease is more common. One of the hallmarks of dementia with Lewy bodies is the fluctuation of cognitive functioning. Often, a patient may function well one day and on the next be totally disengaged, with sudden and profound impairments of mobility, memory and speech. In the case of Mr Dixon, the switch could occur in a matter of minutes. He might be able to stand up and take a few steps at one moment and collapse at the next. 'Living his everyday roller coaster of dementia with Lewy bodies', to quote one carer, Mr Dixon was observed to switch often between different modalities of consciousness, leading to a precarious existence between what is real and what is dream-like.

Once, I witnessed how the unpredictable switch between sleeping and waking, over which he had absolutely no conscious control, could overtake Mr Dixon suddenly. 'Is this a dream? Where am I?' Slowly turning his head and upper body towards his right, Mr Dixon asked this question to Mrs Almond, the resident sitting beside him on the couch. With her smile frozen, Mrs Almond stared at him with her mouth half-open. After a few seconds, Mrs Almond looked across Mr Dixon to me, sitting on the left side of the couch. Just one moment ago, Mr Dixon was sitting comfortably with Mrs Almond and me watching a gourmet food and travel programme on television. He was amiable, smiling and chatting with apparent ease and pleasure. One moment later, he looked confused, distant and frail. Caught by surprise, Mrs Almond was speechless and looked puzzled. Sensing the sudden change in him, I responded in a low, gentle voice: 'Mr Dixon, you are not in a dream. You are in the lounge with Mrs Almond and me.' With a blank face, he sank back, dropped his head to his chest and fell asleep. On such occasions, staff usually let Mr Dixon sleep without disturbing him. 'Don't wake him up,' they said. 'He hits you if you wake him up. Don't worry. He will be fine when he wakes up on his own.' Being woken up might have exacerbated his confusion between dream and reality. Perhaps this was the explanation for Mr Dixon's extreme aggression.

His question 'Is this a dream?' might indicate his disorientation when in the state between being awake and asleep. One minute he was actively engaging in the conversation with Mrs Almond and me, and then he quickly became unresponsive and unaware of the people around him. Mr Dixon's experience illustrates that any mode of being-in-the-world is a becoming. The uncertainty, ambiguity and unpredictability of the present and the future become an embedded feature of becoming-in-the-world. Between becoming-moving – active and engaged – and staying still – asleep and inactive – the everyday life of Mr Dixon was lived in a rhizomatic way like 'an amassing of middles amidst an array of multidirectional movement' (Sellers and Honan 2007: 146). In his abrupt falling asleep, Mr Dixon seemed to have closed up within himself in a state of serenity, stillness and solitude.

Unlike residents with impaired but relatively stable cognitive functioning, Mr Dixon experienced fluctuations of cognition, speech, memory and mobility. The most difficult part of caring for Mr Dixon was due to the fact that most of the time he lived in altered lifeworlds of his own, to which other people were denied access. On his bad days, Mr Dixon inhabited a hostile and threatening lifeworld due to his sensory impairments, meaning that the messages his senses sent to his brain were not being interpreted properly. Mr Dixon could become upset if unexpectedly moved or even touched by carers during assisted transfer. He could get irritated when carers dressed him after a shower. I saw that he looked insecure whenever having to stand upright and easily became panicky if he tipped off balance. He also suffered from visuospatial difficulties, including inability to distinguish left from right, to follow directions, or to recognize objects. He seemed to have no awareness of his body in relation to other things and persons in the environment. He would stop suddenly in front of a rug because his impaired depth perception might lead him to perceive a rug as a hole in the floor.

In biomedical explanations, dementia affects perception because the disease slowly destroys the parts of the brain that are responsible for converting sensory input into meaningful information. Mr Dixon often said things that suggested he had a different idea of 'reality', or sense of what is really going on, from people around him. Staff frequently talked about him 'seeing stuff no one else could see'. One day he was seen waving his arms over his plate of fish and chips: he was hallucinating and believed there was a strange young man in his room eating his lunch. On another occasion, he looked frightened and asked the carer walking into his room: 'Did you see that black pussy cat in my bed?' When she told him that no cat was there, he reacted angrily, and told her to go and have her eyes checked.

He was also paranoid and had delusions. One day he became convinced that an impostor was pretending to be his daughter – stealing all his money and allowing strangers (staff) to live in his house. He wanted to call the police and get them to remove the unwelcome strangers from his room. Delusions were manifestations of Mr Dixon's worst fears; sadly, he saw them as facts.

Cognitive impairments affect perception as well as memory and cognition. When perception is affected, it becomes very hard to make sense of the world, not to mention have a sense of home. Mr Dixon, once a head engineer of a big mining company, an amateur helicopter pilot, a vibrant sportsman, a loved father and grandfather, and a friend to many people, slowly became, to use his close friend's words, 'a shadow of himself'. For nursing home residents like Mr Dixon, their lives are worlds apart from that of people around them. There is little room for togetherness or shared understanding. Scared, confused, sad and delusional, they are struggling to make connections they once made so easily and to have a sense of control amidst the chaos that they live daily.

Having said that, dementia with Lewy bodies does differ from other dementias in the occasional window of clarity it offers, where an affected person can appear to be alert, verbal and mobile. Mr Dixon had days like this. He looked quite different on such occasions, with his eyebrows raised cheerfully and his deep facial lines smoothed out. People were often surprised to see him out of his own room, sitting in a wheelchair or walking with staff assistance (with another carer pushing a wheelchair behind in anticipation of any emergency). 'Oh, he's awake now. He looks a lot brighter,' one visitor said about Mr Dixon. Staff referred to these days as his 'better days', and on those days he would talk to them, follow their instructions for transfers, show understanding, be helpful and accept help. I could feel a sense of relief when carers were able to assist Mr Dixon with transfer from his comfort chair into a wheelchair with apparent ease. They would say: 'We are in luck with Mr Dixon today. This is one of his better days.' On one such day, they wheeled him to the lounge to join a group of residents doing stretching exercises, led by the occupational therapist. Sitting with his glass of lemonade on the tea table, Mr Dixon looked relaxed and placid. He even started a conversation with the elderly lady sitting next to him.

On his better days, Mr Dixon was seen by people around him as 'coming back with more sense': seeing the world as it appears to others and responding to it as people usually do. He noticed when a carer approached in response to his attempt to rise from a chair; he knew what to do when staff brought his walker in front of him; he put a firm grip on the handlebars of his walker, and he leaned forward to stand up. On such occasions, we could say that Mr Dixon and other material things and persons 'corresponded' (Ingold 2017: 16). In corresponding, the world becomes real again; it makes sense in and through sight, hearing and touch. He could respond with appropriate gestures; for example, reaching out to grip a helping hand. When he conversed with someone sitting next to him, Mr Dixon was expressing a sense of rightness of being with others and that the world was once more a right place to be. Being just for a while free from the shadow of dementia, Mr Dixon could talk in full sentences and move confidently by himself around the nursing home.

Those days or hours could not last: usually without warning, and far too soon, he would again become unresponsive and withdraw into his solitude.

Yet, as long as the drive to move flowed through him, Mr Dixon was able to rediscover some sense of control in and through his movement and through corresponding with other people and things in his environment.

Caring for residents with cognitive and movement fluctuations, like those of Mr Dixon, poses a challenge to providers and caregivers. There were limitations to Mr Dixon's ability to move, particularly when he was in his somnolent state. But on his better days, Mr Dixon could become alert and exhibit an obvious desire to move. There were also potential benefits for him to continue walking. Living in the tension between walking and not walking, Mr Dixon could be assisted to walk at those times when he experienced heightened awareness, cognition and mobility, if and when his attempt to move was met by a right assemblage of care. This happened when carers noticed his changed demeanour and responded to his attempts to move by offering assistance.

For residents who live in the tension between walking and not walking, continuing movement depends on their connecting and corresponding with the bodies of other staff and assistive technologies, such as walking aids. But in order for these assemblages of people and things to come together and motivate residents to walk, carers must be hyper-attentive to the shifting states of residents' minds and bodies. Adjustments to those assemblages need to be constantly made if residents are to feel right and to walk well. An assemblage of care is right if it works to produce the movements a resident wishes to make. This means that a right assemblage of care cannot be easily nailed down in care plans. Just as good days differ from bad days, what is right for a resident will change according to the vicissitudes of bodies and situations. Assemblages of care require constant 'tinkering' from one moment to the next (Mol, Moser and Pols 2010).

## What Is the 'Right' Care for Mr Dixon?

This book has so far tried to show that how each individual resident experiences their movements is embodied and situated, and thus unique to them. Bodily impairments are both constitutive and differentiating in defining how residents can walk and continue to walk. Unlike Mrs Sage, who could walk freely on her own, or Mr Harris, who could hardly walk at all without his Parkinson's medication and staff assistance, Mr Dixon experienced constant wild fluctuations of mobility and cognition. He was able to walk unaided at one moment but then was prone to collapsing the next. As all of this could happen in the blink of eye, Mr Dixon needed an assemblage of care that was responsive to his shifting states. A male carer who had previously worked in a hospital once told me that, ideally,

Mr Dixon should be cared for with one-on-one supervision so that he could be promptly attended to when he attempted to move. Or, as another care worker mentioned to me, residents with similar impairments to Mr Dixon could be organized to sit together in a designated area with one staff member supervising and calling for help from other staff whenever any of them attempted to stand and walk.

But the carer went on to point out an obvious problem: 'We don't have the level of funding that hospitals do.' Rostering extra staff in order to respond as needed to residents who exhibit spontaneous movement means increased expense and decreased efficiency. Let's also consider that for the care management team (mostly doctors and nurses) in the facility these spontaneous movements were not 'windows of opportunity' for residents to walk. On the contrary, those episodes were seen as risks to be managed and mitigated.

Surveillance of his movements to prevent falls was the main objective of Mr Dixon's carers. To help achieve that objective, a sensor mat was prescribed for Mr Dixon as part of his Fall Prevention Plan. When Mr Dixon stepped on the sensor mat, the multisensory – audio, visual and textual – alarm system was activated to notify staff of his movements so they could attend to him. The sensor mat thus facilitated sensory extensions that linked Mr Dixon's movements to those of his carers. How carers were expected to respond to the sensor mat alarm was made explicit, documented in staff work procedures and reinforced every now and then by the registered nurse on duty.

After becoming familiar with the alarm system, an observer could easily tell Mr Dixon's bad days from his good days. On the bad days, the monitor screen constantly turned red and displayed his room number. Staff were then frequently summoned from other activities to check on Mr Dixon. But carers are responsible for routinely delivering care to all residents in the unit. So the bad days for Mr Dixon – seen from the staffing point of view – were also bad days for carers working in the unit. The situation with Mr Dixon was like the example provided in Chapter 3, in which the extra assistance provided to Mr Harris meant an extra burden for carers. In relation to Mr Dixon, as well as the heavy load of their routine work, staff had to make time (that they did not have) to respond promptly to each episode when he tried to move from his chair. By using the adjective 'bad', carers were indicating their own stress in coping with the constant attempts of Mr Dixon to get out of his chair. Staff told me that they felt 'stretched', running from resident to resident on those bad days, while also trying to reduce the risk of residents falling and the incidence of residents becoming aggressive.

In attending to Mr Dixon as per standard fall prevention procedure, staff usually told Mr Dixon to sit back into his chair while they reset the sensor mat and then rushed away to attend to other competing priorities and scheduled care tasks. When staff did attend to Mr Dixon, they seemed dismissive of his desire to stand up and attempt to move. In fact, they disregarded his efforts by encouraging him to stay seated. So the sensor mat effectively prevents residents from standing up and walking. Carers explained that, from their point of view, residents in the later stages of dementia may 'forget' that they can't keep their balance when standing or walking.

Although a resident might feel an urge to stand up and walk, they may not realize that to walk safely they need assistance. As shown in the example of Mrs Sage, ongoing staff supervision and prompt assistance are crucial for residents with cognitive impairments to keep safe while walking. If staff were able to attend to Mr Dixon whenever the alarm went off and assist him to move, the use of a sensor mat, as an innovative assistive technology, could play an important role in delivering the 'right' care for him. Creating an assemblage of care that assists residents like Mr Dixon to move is critical to their becoming at ease in their unpredictable bodies. In Part II of this book, I foreground the topic of care to critically examine the different ways of doing care in residential care facilities. I explore the many ways that residents may be prevented from moving in the name of care and, conversely, how the right care can enable and support residents' innermost drive to move.

# PART II
## Care

During my fieldwork, the care management team in one of the facilities started an initiative in which residents were invited to nominate a staff member to be the Star Employee of the Month. One staff member would be selected from the nominees and identified with praise in the facility's newsletter. Once, in the lounge area, a resident pointed to the carer's photo in the newsletter and said, 'I nominated Maureen. She is a good carer. She does care!' Another carer, who was standing nearby responded by saying, 'Mrs Joyce, I do the same for you as Maureen. We all do the same care work. So do you think that I don't care?' Mrs Joyce looked at the care worker and said, 'That's right; you all do the same care work, but differently. That's how I feel about it.' In a chat with Mrs Joyce following that conversation, she told me that although the carers generally do the same things for her, like showering, dressing and grooming, some carers can make things easier for her while others may leave her feeling distressed. She explained: 'It doesn't feel right when some carers help me to stand up. They don't let me do it myself. They just drag me up and pull me forward. I feel terrible when they rush me through the morning routine.'

Conversations like these illustrate the different, and at times contested, understandings and experiences of care in nursing homes. Care work may be a task performed by care workers, but it does not necessarily lead to residents feeling cared for. Mrs Joyce makes a distinction between two modes of care work: staff doing work vs staff doing work with care. Both modes involve embodied labour: the former prioritizes the need to get a job done, often quickly, leading to feelings of being rushed and roughly handled, while the latter prioritizes affective engagement, creating a feeling of being assisted with care. Maureen knew how to do her work with care, and she made Mrs Joyce feel respected and comfortable when she did it. This was apparent to me when I saw her assisting Mrs Joyce and allowing her to take the lead in her movements and transfer of positions.

In this part, I want to explore the disjuncture between *how care is done* as work and *how care is felt* by residents. Care work that is itemized in work procedures, such as responding to a sensor mat alarm, as described in

Chapter 4, may or may not contribute to residents' *feelings* of being cared for. What staff need to do in providing hands-on care – for example, showering or giving a massage – is related to broader issues of care; these need assessment and planning, which in turn regulate hands-on care and how residents experience it. As I will show in the first section of Chapter 5, what staff perform as work is shaped by multiple and often contesting discourses, perspectives and notions of care. The everyday intersection, contestation and negotiation involved in care practices may make nursing home care, as Perkinson claims in her ethnographic study, indeed, 'multiple realities of care' (2003: 258) for people who either live or work in that environment.

With a focus on tasks, schedules and efficiency, 'doing work' may make staff insensitive to residents' wounds and weeping skins and become affectively disengaged. They might push, pull or grasp a person, inattentive to how the force of their fingertips may cause pain or leave bruises. At meal times, they are unlikely to make the time and effort to sufficiently prepare residents with late-stage dementia for the event of eating. Conversely, the mode of doing work *with care* foregrounds residents' personal comfort, with staff attentive to where they place their hands, and with what force, when rolling a resident, or how careful they might need to be when inserting a spoon into their mouths. Approaching residents' experiences through sensory analysis (Dennis 2018) leads to the realization that asymmetrical power relations (Martin, Myers and Viseu 2015: 626) are always entailed in daily care delivery.

Doing work with care, as Mrs Joyce indicated, can never be assumed; it is contingent on changing perspectives and circumstances. More than once, staff working with Maureen complained about her 'talking too much with residents' and being 'fussy with tasks like manual handling or feeding', which, from their perspective, slowed down morning routines.

In the contested cultural space and complex lifeworld of the nursing home, approaching service provision with an attention to *working with care* is to direct attention to the neglected experiences of residents and the uncompensated 'doings with care' performed by personal care workers. It points to the contextual effect of sociopolitically contingent arrangements of care and the asymmetry of power. As will be shown, residents' bodily experiences and staff efforts to respond to their needs and wishes are elided in the existing aged care system. Accordingly, this work seeks to explore 'how these arrangements of care and power might be otherwise' (Martin, Myers and Viseu 2015: 628) in a reconfiguration of aged care.

# 5 CARE AS MULTIPLICITIES

## Deconstructing Nursing Home Care

In nursing homes, care is centrally organized. But how it is understood and enacted varies from person to person, be they management, clinicians, carers, residents or family. In this chapter, I want to write about care in nursing homes as multiplicities, examining how tensions between care practices and policies become embodied in the movements of residents. I explore contradictions and contestations of care by extending assemblages of care beyond the bodies and material things that are involved in daily care activities to the care policies, plans and assessments that construct and itemize care delivery. As I will show, care as it is currently practised in residential aged care can actually reduce possibilities for residents to become at home in that environment. To create right assemblages of care for residents with impaired mobility and cognition, we need a combination of innovative ideas and technologies.

It is important to note that the contesting forces, embedded in the government funding scheme and the cultural imperatives of medicine, economy and domesticity, interplay in rhizomatic ways, intersecting and parting in complex ways, rather than simply operating alongside each other. According to Deleuze, we can hold in tension multiple interplays and paradoxes and examine them as multiplicities: different assemblages of things, persons, processes, discourses and practices will emerge and actualize into movements, against a background of ever-changing circumstances.

Deleuze's concept of multiplicity is useful for developing a new analysis on the interplay of the multiple processes and forces that constitute the medicalized treatments and daily living support that nursing home residents need. In this section, I will draw on the example of Mrs Joyce to deconstruct nursing home care into its multiple assemblages: making assessments, care planning and scheduling of routine activities . In so doing, I aim to reveal how care is variously understood, articulated and practised in the nursing homes.

### *Assessments: Constructing Care Needs*

In Australia, an overwhelming proportion of elderly people are admitted into residential aged care due to acute medical conditions that lead to their hospitalization. Mrs Joyce was transferred by ambulance to a hospital emergency department with a cracked femur after having a fall while going to the toilet in the night. After spending five weeks in hospital, her bone crack was stable, and she was allowed to walk and weight-bear as pain permitted. However, she could no longer take care of herself independently. She needed someone to assist her with all daily activities. Older Australians are supported to live independently in their own homes through the home care packages programme. This programme is funded by the federal government and provided through a coordinated mix of services that can include: help with household tasks, equipment (such as walking frames), minor home modifications, personal care, clinical care such as nursing, and allied health services such as physiotherapy. To be eligible to receive these government-funded care services, an older person needs approval from an Aged Care Assessment Team (ACAT). Staff in the hospital referred Mrs Joyce for an ACAT assessment to test her eligibility, and if eligible, the level of home care she could be approved for. ACAT is a government unit responsible for carrying out assessments of older people's needs, using the Aged Care Funding Instrument (ACFI). The resulting assessment is referred to as an Aged Care Client Record.

In the case of Mrs Joyce, she was assessed as not suitable for a home care package. Even with the highest level (Level 4) of home care support, Mrs Joyce could no longer live alone at home because of her complex care needs. Her husband had died from bowel cancer five years before. Her daughter had moved overseas with her family, and her son was interstate working in a mining company. They both made regular phone calls and sent her birthday and Christmas cards but neither of them could do anything to help with her daily living. Before her hospital admission, Mrs Joyce often sought help with house maintenance or financial issues from Helen, her niece, who also lives in Adelaide.

As Mrs Joyce could no longer manage at home without help, she was approved for entry into high-level residential aged care. Residential aged care can be offered as either permanent or short-term care. Short-term care in an aged care home is called residential respite care and is designed to give family carers a break for a limited period of time. In the case of Mrs Joyce, however, she entered the nursing home as a permanent resident. Only those elderly people who are assessed as in need of high-level care and therefore eligible for entry are admitted into permanent residential aged care. As more people now choose to age in their own homes, permanent residential aged care is increasingly focused on catering for people when they are nearing their end of life. In fact, the average age of admission to residential aged care is now 84.6 years (Department of Health 2019). As a needs-based funding tool, ACFI assessments are conducted to allocate government funding to cover senior Australians' most up-to-date care needs. The ACFI affects how elderly Australians are supported with daily living by differentiating (through eligibility assessment) and categorizing (into different levels) elderly people into the aged care system as per the type and level of care best suited to their needs.

On her admission day, I joined Mrs Joyce and her niece Helen in their meeting with Julie, the admission nurse. Sitting at the side of her hospital bed, Mrs Joyce looked lost, sad and exhausted. Julie seemed to understand how Mrs Joyce felt on her first day in a nursing home and tried to comfort her. 'Don't worry, Mrs Joyce,' Julie said, and added: 'In four weeks, we will work out a care plan for you. Every detail of your daily living will be discussed and covered. For now, we only need to work out some basics so that staff are prepared when they come to help you.'

Julie then started asking questions about how Mrs Joyce undertook everyday activities: for example, bathing, dressing, grooming, toilet use, feeding, transfers, walking and climbing stairs. Mrs Joyce told Julie that she had gone through the same list of questions with another nurse in the hospital. 'What you had in the hospital was an eligibility assessment,' Julie replied. 'What we are doing now is part of the admission assessment.' Julie continued to explain to Mrs Joyce and Helen that the results of the admission assessments would indicate her level of functional ability and degree of independence, which would provide a picture of her immediate care needs. As previously mentioned, eligibility for government funding was the essential element for Mrs Joyce to enter a residential facility. On admission into a nursing home, more comprehensive assessments are conducted to further allocate human (staff shift time, attention and assistance) and material (aiding devices, assistive equipment and technology) resources to each individual resident within the co-funding scheme of government subsidies and residents' own financial contribution.

Julie then used the Barthel ADL Index to measure the performance of Mrs Joyce on the Activities of Daily Living (ADLs). As Julie went through the questions with her, Mrs Joyce told Julie that she could 'manage' on her own well when she was not in pain. Julie then asked Mrs Joyce to show her how she got herself out of bed. Mrs Joyce, on trying to demonstrate, could not manage this. When she tried to lift her buttocks up from the edge of the bed, she just fell back. Julie scored 5 points for both the activity of 'transfer' and 'walking' for Mrs Joyce, which meant that she needed some help to do both activities. She scored 0 points for the activity of 'climbing stairs' as she was unable to do this, even with the aid of her walking stick. Based on the results of this initial assessment, 'one staff for physical assistance with transfer and locomotion' was temporarily assigned to Mrs Joyce.

In aged care service provision, residents' walking, making transfers from one position to another, eating, drinking, showering, dressing, grooming and toileting are classified as the Activities of Daily Living (ADLs). As shown in the Barthel ADL Index that Julie used to measure Mrs Joyce's performance, 'care needs' of a resident include whether the resident needs staff supervision or assistance with making the necessary movements involved for the daily living activities, such as transfer of positions from lying to sitting or sitting to standing. In this sense, the term 'care needs' refers to the extent of staff assistance that is necessary for supporting residents to move. Take Julie's prescription for Mrs Joyce as an example: 'One staff physical assistance with transfer and locomotion' is the ACFI term for a specific caregiving activity. In the ACFI User Guide, activities are defined as 'the action steps to meet a care need'. The care need of a resident is 'informed by an assessment' (Department of Health and Ageing 2013: 3).

Care needs assessment also relates to another two components of nursing home care: government funding and care planning. The government funding scheme regulates financial support to care service providers, who organize daily service delivery through care planning. The logic of the ACFI as a medicalized funding instrument is to match the resident's needs with the provided care so that what is conceived as lacking in the resident's bodily capacity can be provided through the caregivers' prescribed action steps. The key to matching care with 'needs' is, as Mrs Joyce's example shows, to assess residents' experiences and demonstrated abilities. Then, how they can or cannot move can be described quantitatively so that care – in the form of a walking aid or staff attention and assistance – can be matched and prescribed. So assessments are done to determine how staff assistance is to be provided in its varied forms and styles, in order to support residents' movements and engagement in daily activities.

Within four weeks of her admission into the care facility, staff had completed all the comprehensive assessments on Mrs Joyce's care needs. The assessments covered her medical history, diagnosis, ongoing medication and treatment, as well as her life history, family and cultural background, habits and preferences. The culture of medicalization in aged care services is one in which an increasing number of the older person's bodily processes are subject to what Foucault (2012) described as 'the clinical gaze'. This means that bodily movements, senses and feelings of elderly people are all judged in terms of medical observations, diagnosis and treatment: the aged become the diseased. In nursing home jargon, the older person's movements become the nurse's 'transfer', the older person's walking becomes the physiotherapist's 'ambulation', the older person's food becomes the nutritionist's 'diet', the older person's eccentricities become the staff's 'behaviours', and the older person's life becomes the institutional 'record' (Stafford 2003a). As an organized system of linguistic terminology, medicine provides the regulating norms for thinking and doing in the nursing home.

### *'Care Planning': Entanglement of Meanings and Processes*

Providing tailored support and assistance to each individual resident poses a challenge to aged care service providers. The challenge comes from the complexity of allocating limited human and material resources to each resident according to their needs. As shown in the previous subsection, planning is a key component for organizing material and human resources into daily care practices within the constraints of the government funding scheme. In the sector of residential aged care, it is mandated that a service provider must conduct a clinical process of care planning. Resources, such as walking aids, equipment and staff assistance, are allocated in the form of a written care plan and then implemented in routinized activities of daily living.

Routine care practice involves an up-to-date care plan for each person, one that is required to reflect the current health status of the person and respect their individual personhood. In the case of Mrs Joyce, mobility was a key aspect of her care plan. After the physiotherapist reviewed her medical history and conducted a mobility care assessment using the Physical Mobility Scale, he recorded that Mrs Joyce needed a 4-wheeled walker and staff assistance with transfers. In light of her hospitalization, Mrs Joyce was also identified as at risk of falling at night. A Fall Prevention Plan was therefore created for Mrs Joyce, including having a sensor mat at her bedside.

The discourse of person-centred care has had increasing consequences for daily care practices, especially in regard to care planning. With an emphasis on providing individualized care, information about family, education and employment histories, interests, hobbies, habits and preferences is now collected in admission assessments, considered in care planning, and used to shape daily care delivery. An individualized care plan is thought to help the resident to adapt and adjust to their nursing home life through establishing and following a daily routine that reflects their needs and preferences. After familiarizing themselves with Mrs Joyce's care plan, morning shift carers knew to unplug her sensor mat first thing after handover, and in turn Mrs Joyce learned not to get up on her own, which would activate the alarm. Instead, she would wait in bed for staff assistance with transferring her position ready for walking. After a long night of lying in bed,

Mrs Joyce often felt stiff and in pain from her neck, back and shoulders. While she was used to having an evening shower at home, she found the new routine of the morning shower soothing and refreshing. Knowing what to expect – warm water on her aches and pains – enabled Mrs Joyce to feel at ease and to look forward to the new day.

Care services are divided into Mobility Care and Fall Prevention because the two categories are funded differently. For Mrs Joyce, these care services – which are jointly delivered and included the use of a 4-wheeled walker, staff assistance with transfers and a sensor mat to alert staff of her movements at night – created a right assemblage of care for her to mobilize as she wished and to feel comfortable at home in the nursing home.

Nevertheless, itemizing residents' conditions and needs into separate categories in residents' care plan and using ACFI criteria to allocate and deliver services do not always lead to a right assemblage of care. For example, a massage from a registered nurse or physiotherapist was correctly prescribed in Mrs Joyce's Pain Management Plan but was not always delivered, for reasons that will be explained later.

Treatment for pain is categorized in the ACFI as addressing residents' Complex Care Needs. Residents were widely assessed for pain after this category of Complex Care Needs was added to the ACFI. Staff chose to use the Pain Assessment In Advanced Dementia (PAINAD) scale to assess Mrs Joyce even though she did not have a medical diagnosis of dementia. The PAINAD assessment shows higher sensibility and validity, as the instrument is observational and does not depend on a resident recounting their experience of pain. Staff explained to me that they used the PAINAD assessment for Mrs Joyce because although pain is experienced by many residents, some residents tend to downplay their experience of pain, and difficulty, as shown when Mrs Joyce said that she could manage her change of position from sitting to standing when she could not.

Mrs Joyce did experience pain and usually received a daily massage on her neck, shoulders and lower back after her morning shower. Massage is part of the Activities of Daily Living (ADLs), performed daily by personal carers. After her pain assessment, Mrs Joyce was prescribed 20-minute massage sessions administered weekly by either a registered nurse or a physiotherapist. Daily and weekly massages belong to different categories. The weekly sessions are part of the Pain Management Plan to address the resident's Complex Care Needs (a category in the ACFI). Extra funding is provided by the federal government to service providers for meeting residents' Complex Care Needs. However, a daily after-shower massage is not a government-funded service item. While showering is funded under the category of Personal Care Needs, an after-shower massage is provided as per the resident's request and preference, with the agreement of staff.

The ACFI is not designed to guide day-to-day service provision but to assess 'core care needs' of residents for the purpose of allocating funding to residential aged care providers. What residents need in terms of support and assistance with their day-to-day living may exceed what can be categorized and covered using the ACFI. Mrs Joyce, of course, knew nothing about the categories or the funding. She just knew she enjoyed a relaxing massage right after her morning shower. A right assemblage of care to treat Mrs Joyce's pain would have included a daily massage session after her shower. However, as part of the sequence of activities between showering and dressing, the time allowed for massage was often cut short by carers, as time was almost always tight. As for the weekly prescribed pain management massage, Mrs Joyce asked, what is the point in getting undressed for a massage in the middle of the day? While she was expected to benefit from the 20-minute weekly massage, she often missed out on this session because she was taking part in social activities, like a Cafe & Chat session.

Among aged care researchers, the written care plan is widely believed to orient staff to deliver individualized care, maintain the continuity of care and promote team communication. Yet, what is often disregarded is the financial consideration embedded in the process of care planning and documenting. To maximize financial support from government funding, residents' care needs are constructed within the ACFI conceptual framework so that services provided can be accounted for and hence funded by the government. It is important for staff to do the paperwork: to document what they do for residents; for example, by completing a Bowels Chart or by filling in numbers on a Food and Fluid Intake Form. 'It is essential to get the work documented if the work is done,' the care manager emphasized. If the work is not documented, it is regarded as not done, even if it has actually been done. Documentation of care work makes staff accountable for their work for purposes such as accreditation or for funding approval. A tick of the box for Weekly Massage on Mrs Joyce's Pain Management Record Sheet was directly linked to the facility's claim for extra subsidies to meet Mrs Joyce's Complex Care Need of managing pain. ACFI thus possesses in written form a defining power in how care is inscribed, funded and practised in nursing homes. Extra staff time can flow from the extra funding, which is why a massage shift by a registered nurse was created to deliver weekly massage sessions to residents after the Complex Care Needs category was created.

The invisible but overarching and decisive impact of the funding scheme on residents' care planning may lead to unexpected consequences. It has been reported that staff did not refer to care plans in delivering care, as they often thought care plans were not meaningful for delivering individualized care (Yun-Hee et al. 2013). It was also reported in a Norwegian study that even when residents were given person-centred care, their care needs were not reflected in their care plans (Sandvoll, Kristoffersen and Hauge 2012). My own fieldwork observations suggest that staff are more likely to be oriented by local work/task sheets (a schedule of tasks to be carried out within the time frame of a shift) rather than by the resident's care plan. Residents' habits and preferences are often updated day to day, service by service, on the worksheets with no reference to the care plan. If we compare what is planned (what should be done) and documented (what is done) with the actual playing out of events in real time, situations and relationships are far more nuanced than care plans imply. Life 'on the ground' in nursing homes comprises caregiving as multiplicities: the coming together, playing out and intertwining of many components, such as government funding schemes, care needs assessments, care planning and daily care delivery. They form different assemblages of care; some are productive in meeting residents' needs while others fail to do so. It is in daily routinized activities that different assemblages of care are enacted and connections between residents and supportive other material things and persons are actualized. It is in this space that tensions between contesting forces become evident in and through residents' 'becoming and unbecoming moving' as we will see below.

## *Routines: The Actual Play Out of Events 'on the Floor'*

As the brief account of Mrs Joyce's morning routine demonstrates, how elderly people adjust to the institutional way of life in a nursing home is affected by how staff assistance is provided. This includes establishing and following everyday personal routines, such as sleeping/waking, eating and washing, activities that involve both residents' own efforts and staff assistance within scheduled time slots. Initial care plans are mostly made after consultation with residents and their significant others to reflect their own interests and preferences at the beginning of their residency. As time goes on, daily activities become routinized through everyday practice. As Chapter 1 demonstrated, using the example of Mrs Casey, her personal routines were closely associated with a feeling of being at ease and in harmony with the facility's operations.

Personal carers are usually allocated to a unit to attend to all the residents living there. In the care facility where Mrs Joyce lives, four morning shift carers attend to 28 residents in the unit, all of whom have various physical and cognitive impairments.[1] Staff either work in pairs or on their own, depending on the level of care needed by residents (e.g. a 1- or 2-person physical assist with transfer). The allocated personal care time for each resident in the morning is around 20 minutes, and this includes toileting, showering, dressing, grooming, making the bed and cleaning the room. Aside from general tasks like showering and dressing, personal care staff also need to perform some specific tasks (in the category of 'technical needs') for each resident, such as 'saline eyelid scrub to both eyes', 'alcohol wipes between toes' or 'Tubigrip to both legs, toe to knee'.[2] According to agency staff, in comparison with other care facilities, this resident to staff ratio (7:1) was quite reasonable, as a few residents were classed as 'self-care' with transfers and walking.[3] In a Canadian residential aged care facility, one carer was reported to undertake ADLs for nine residents with physical disability and cognitive impairment on day shift while two staff members cared for 27 residents at night. Those caregivers described the workload as 'overwhelming' and 'insane' (DeForge et al. 2011: 419).

The 20-minute per resident time frame in the morning is an integral part of the overarching institutional routine – a structuring of time slots regulating the collective ways and styles of work organization. Characteristic of institutional routines are the temporal markers placed on the commencing and completing of certain tasks; for example, serving lunch from 12 PM to 1 PM, administering medication at mealtimes, assisting residents in the morning from 7 AM to 11 AM, etc. Serving as what Zerubavel (1979) described as 'temporal reference frameworks', institutional routines affect work performance, in that staff are expected to complete a list of certain tasks at a certain rhythm, speed and tempo and within a particular time slot in order to synchronize with co-workers and staff working in other departments, such as catering or housekeeping.

How care staff are organized by the institutional routines affects the extent to which they can assist residents with their daily activities. The time allocated to assist each resident (e.g. 20 minutes) is set, and there are always some residents waiting to be assisted; however, staff must keep the pace moving briskly as they move from one resident to the next. It is worth remembering that while staff can adjust pace by speeding up if necessary, elderly residents move at their own individual pace, due to their bodily conditions, and cannot be rushed to move faster. When staff face time pressures to finish work with one resident, they may look for shortcuts. So, for example, rather than assisting the resident to walk using their walker, they are more likely to use a wheelchair, to speed up the transportation. But in that replacement the resident may not feel 'right' – they are restrained from making their own movements and lose their feeling of control and connectedness in and through walking. In this sense, the institutional power of the nursing home is exerted directly upon their bodies by either allowing them to connect and move or by restraining them.

Part and parcel of the institutionalization of people living and working in nursing homes is that they come to regard institutional routines as the normal and accustomed structure of daily functioning. Bland cites Savishinsky to point out that a clockwork schedule of meals, medications, therapies, bathing and shift changeovers constitutes a rigid framework of routine care practice (1991: 119 as in Bland 2007: 942). The institutional care practice routine is often criticized for its emphasis on efficiency. In her study of nursing home residents' experience of comfort, Bland concluded that: 'Cultural practices, such as care delivery routines, were so entrenched they had become the taken-for-granted way of functioning' and 'are driven more by a desire for organizational efficiency than the comfort of residents' (2003: 187).

Nevertheless, with new government initiatives in Australia emphasizing the person-centred care approach, carers have recently received training on how to provide more flexible support and assistance to residents that acknowledges personal needs and preferences. As I observed in my fieldwork, mealtimes were sometimes extended to suit an individual resident's condition and situation and shower routines could be negotiable, depending on the availability of time, resources and staff.

How each staff member organizes their daily work is often contested and must be negotiated, not only according to residents' habits and preferences but also to acknowledge those 'background expectations' that require staff to constantly perform 'the act of time management' (Adam 1995: 42). In this sense, *staff routines* can be understood as to some extent a justified stable structure for the ADLs to be carried out in a timely, labour-saving and straightforward manner to suit both residents' personal routines and institutional ones. Some veteran carers had the reputation of being able to, as the managers and nurses said, 'know their work' to 'get the work done' and 'know their residents' in providing individualized care.

In the entangled processes of daily care delivery, unexpected events may disturb the routinized work plan and expose the complex interplay of contesting forces and discourses, including the overarching institutional routines, the staff roster and allocation system, and the discourses of efficiency and person-centred care. In one facility, I took the opportunity to record the number of resident call bells I heard on two consecutive mornings, to explore how, in a situation of staff shortage, the *absence* of staff assistance, which is a key component of daily care delivery, may impact on residents' experience.

On the first morning, one care worker did not arrive for his 7 AM to 3 PM shift. As no contracted care staff were available that morning, an agency care worker was booked. Being called in at short notice, the agency worker arrived at 9 AM. That meant that between 7 AM and 9 AM on that morning, instead of having three care workers on the floor, there were only two. The following morning, all three regular care staff (rostered to work for the same shift in the same area) were at work. Kitchen staff routinely started serving breakfast at 8 AM, so a certain number of residents need to be showered and dressed and set up for breakfast before 8 AM. While kitchen staff were serving breakfast in the dining area and sending out breakfast trays into the residents' rooms, the carers were expected to assist residents with their breakfast and feed those residents who could not feed themselves. One care worker short on the floor would mean that some residents would be unattended before and during breakfast. Residents usually ring their call bell to alert staff that they need help. A ring of the call bell indicates a resident's effort to seek staff assistance. Repeated rings of the call bell from the same resident would indicate that staff had failed to respond promptly to the resident's call.

As shown in the data collected, the dramatic increase in the total number of resident call bells being rung, and the pattern of repetitive calls, indicates a gap between residents' need for staff assistance and its provision. There was a dramatic increase of residents ringing call bells when there were only two carers on the floor (19 calls compared to 7 for the next morning). Importantly, one resident made four calls in the span of one and half hours, on that morning. What is conveyed by repeated ringing is residents' experiences of frustration and anxiety when they urgently need help but are kept waiting and, in this case, waiting for 90 minutes. In contrast, on the following morning, when there were three regular care staff on the floor, there was not a single recurring call recorded.

Institutional routine care practice is characterized by orchestrated and repeatable patterns of activity enabled by the systematic organization of resources into processes. Care provided to residents in unexpected situations, such as operating with one carer short, will be dependent on the availability of extra resources, such as assistance from nursing staff or kitchen staff. In an ethnographic study conducted in five US nursing homes, Eileen Jackson (1997) noted two kinds of care: routine care prescribed by the institution, and care provided in response to residents' expressed needs, either as requested by the resident (e.g. verbally or using a call bell) or as observed by the caregiver. The former type of care is basic, visible and formal in the institutional setting, while the latter is largely undocumented and informal but pivotal to the residents' wellbeing.

This discussion highlights the dynamic and processual features of routinized activities in institutional settings. In the daily playing out of routinized activities, different forces interplay, compete and negotiate. As my own research shows, walking, for nursing home residents, is a beneficial activity, where material surroundings, living bodies, assessments, daily practices and auditing processes, walking aids and equipment, notional care plans, and unexpected happenings meet, connect and synthesize, often in states of tension in that environment.

## Mapping Care in and through Walking

In the previous section, I drew on the example of Mrs Joyce to expose the various components of nursing home care, including medicalized assessments, care planning, government funding schemes and daily care practices that are prescribed, prescheduled and routinized but rarely actualized as planned. I will now draw on the example of Mr Harris to consider again residents' experiences of walking or not walking in the environment of institutional care. We can map components of care to expose the entangled processes of connecting, overlapping, contesting and competing of elements in different assemblages of care – assemblages that may enable or constrain residents from walking. The central question that I ask in this section is: How do these components articulate and come together to produce a right, or not so right, assemblage of care?

Mr Harris used to walk as much as he wanted when his bodily condition allowed him more time on his feet. With the aid of a 4-wheeled walker, he walked cautiously. Hours and hours of Mr Harris pushing his walker through the corridors, lounge and dining areas, indenting carpeted floors, created pathways of repeated movement. At this stage of his walking, Mr Harris mostly relied on his walking aid for support and stability and could manage with little staff supervision. The ongoing support from his walker, among other material things and persons, was the key component in an assemblage of care that assisted Mr Harris with his irregular, yet safe walking. While both Mrs Sage and Mr Harris 'wandered', in contrast to the high visibility of Mrs Sage, Mr Harris seemed to be almost invisible. Although he had constant encounters with staff, Mr Harris might as well have been invisible to them. Many staff members overtook or walked past him face to face, saying nothing. In their lack of attention, staff appeared to be oblivious to the presence of Mr Harris as he moved. I wondered why Mr Harris drew no staff attention as he walked. When asked, carers explained that, though Mr Harris was in the habit of walking pointlessly, he was *safe* to walk. He appeared to be 'all right' – he was neither disruptive to other residents nor harmful to himself. Unlike the wandering of Mrs Sage, which was challenging to care management and delivery, the walking of Mr Harris posed no danger to himself or people around him. Staff said they would therefore 'leave him to wander'. While Mr Harris walked safely with his walking aid, he was really allowed to walk as he liked. A right assemblage of care for Mr Harris to walk at that time did not require staff assistance.

However, staff awareness of the walking of Mr Harris gradually changed after his frozen gait increasingly affected his walking. Although his sudden halting or acceleration was temporary, his walking became unstable with an increased possibility of falling. Staff attention was increasingly drawn to his walking when it started to look unsafe. From staff paying no attention to Mr Harris' safe walking to increasingly attending to his unsafe walking, staff attention, or to use the ACFI term, 'supervision', became an indispensable element in a right assemblage of care for Mr Harris to walk. It became pivotal to form a new assemblage of care after Mr Harris developed the frozen gait. With this new element of staff supervision, the composition of a right assemblage of care for Mr Harris to walk had changed. The walking of Mr Harris now became staff-supervised walking. It is important to note that there is a difference between a 'staff stand-by' style of supervision, which is an actual funded item and task, and a staff 'keeping an eye on Mr Harris' style of supervision. The latter kind, as Jackson (1997) observed in her study, is an informal practice of carers, which is not funded, and was mostly what Mr Harris received after he developed the frozen gait.

Though staff felt, as they said, 'stretched' by the extra attention paid to the walking of Mr Harris and his need for occasional hands-on help, they managed within their workload to assist Mr Harris to walk safely. There existed, in effect, a tension between what Mr Harris needed – namely, intermittent staff attention and assistance to continue to walk – and what was made available – the unprescribed and unscheduled extra care given through staff informal practice. However, the informal nature of staff assistance that was involved in Mr Harris's walking made it an unstable and precarious component in his assemblage of care.

The confluence of the combined support from Mr Harris's walker, staff engagement and Mr Harris's own efforts to walk was disrupted when his walking deteriorated. More and more often, Mr Harris was seen by staff as struggling to keep his balance and having near-miss fall incidents. Concerned that he might fall over, carers would rush to him with a chair or wheelchair whenever he looked wobbly. They began to feel that their constant assistance to Mr Harris was disruptive to their work routines. Staff assistance is of course the key component not only in a right assemblage of care for Mr Harris to walk but also in *any* assemblage of care if it is to be actualized in the context of assisting residents with daily living. As discussed in the previous section, all personal care workers were assigned with a work/task list – a list of care duties to be carried out in a sequence, within a time frame. They 'ran' from resident to resident to keep themselves on time. Staff tended to foreground routine work rather than residents' movement, in an environment where getting work done and efficiency are prioritized and praised at the organizational level. They also said that it would be 'unfair' to other residents if they could not get other staff to help with a shower or serving breakfast as scheduled, because those carers were assisting Mr Harris. In fact, residents and their families *did* start to complain about carers being unavailable for scheduled care activities, such as showering.

From their point of view, carers felt an overwhelming sense of being overstretched due to stress and exhaustion. They had a duty of care towards Mr Harris to prevent him from having falls and fall-related injuries, while also having a duty of care towards all the other residents in their particular unit. The considerations for residents' safety (legally significant), mobility, hygiene, nutrition and hydration (biomedically vital), and the expectations for staff to be simultaneously caring (morally essential) and efficient (economically important) do not just co-exist; they contest and compete for priority in staff time, attention and energy. Navigating these entanglements of contesting forces and discourses inevitably affects how carers respond to residents' attempted unsafe movements. While carers liked to have a smooth performance of care work, which gave them a sense of ease, they were, in fact, frequently pulled out of the scheduled workflow. In assisting Mr Harris, they felt overwhelmed. The balance between staff engagement and Mr Harris' efforts to walk was broken when the difficulties for Mr Harris to walk safely increased. An increased amount of staff assistance needed to be formally allocated, by means of care planning, to overcome a tension between what was required (care needs) and what was available (care provision) for Mr Harris to walk safely.

Yet, as we saw earlier with the example of Mrs Joyce, while care planning has to organize and allocate human and material resources into daily care delivery, it must work within the constraints of the government co-funding scheme. The component of staff assistance relates not only to residents' care needs (which are often medically constructed) but also to the availability and distribution of funds (which are directed by government policy, investment and financial management of the service provider). In the current Australian aged care system, the component of staff assistance is an itemized service provided with hourly-paid human labour. As staff are rostered and paid for shift work that is counted by hours, the availability of staff assistance is always timed and limited by funding level. 'More money more care,' as one carer said, expressing that the staffing level in a care facility is directly related to the funding level of its residents. So, while staff assistance is understood to be the key component in a right assemblage of care for residents like Mr Harris to walk safely whenever they desire to do so, *how* this component could *function* in an assemblage of care, whether it be formal and consistent, or informal and occasional, leads us to understand care as a *multiplicity* of emergent 'becomings'.

To map the movement and morphosis of staff assistance as multiplicities, let's return to analyse Mr Harris's 'walking/not walking' in more detail. In the context of carers struggling to handle the extra work (remember this is assistance that is *not* in his care plan or funded) and feeling more and more stressed due to his irregular and unsafe walking, they began to *resist* assisting Mr Harris with his walking. They reported their concern about Mr Harris's unsafe walking orally to the registered nurses (RNs) on duty. As supervisors and team leaders, the RNs passed on reports about Mr Harris' unsafe walking to the care management team by writing 'progress notes'. This was done in keeping with the institutional discourse of risk, an important component in care planning, in which a written report is required to seek any change to the status quo. Mr Harris then had a formal assessment of 'risk of fall' (for funding purposes), since the report noted his 'high risk of falling due to impaired balance' (quoted from Mr Harris's progress notes) and that he had a few near-miss falling incidents while unattended. After a high risk of falls was reported, recorded, measured and recognized through assessments, Mr Harris's care plan was amended to address his changed care needs. These were described as walking with staff assistance (mobility care needs) and, significantly, preventing walking while unattended (fall prevention needs). A Mobility Care Plan and a Fall Prevention Plan were then both set up to address these seemingly unrelated needs for care.

Mr Harris's Fall Prevention Plan was created from the understanding that he was no longer fit enough to walk whenever he liked with his wheelie walker and that it would be better for him to sit rather than to walk while unattended. Carers attending to him took away his walker, replaced it with a sensor mat and sat him in a chair. To prevent him from walking while unattended, his walker was kept out of his reach. His walker was clearly *not* a component in this new assemblage of care, which was based on fall prevention. Meanwhile, as a key component of his new Mobility Care Plan, Mr Harris was prescribed a '2-staff-assisted daily walking routine' after he was restrained from walking on his own. His use of the walker and other elements, including the timed consumption of Parkinson's medication and allocated staff time, could now be organized into fixed temporal, spatial and relational structures of a staff-assisted walking routine so that he could walk safely.

As shown in the example of Mr Harris, the discourse of risk works to break open a closed structure – an assemblage of care that could assist Mr Harris with walking more often but not safely – by taking away the walking aid and stopping unscheduled staff assistance. This solution curtailed his walking considerably. The discourse of risk also worked to arrange a new assemblage of care for him based on risk-oriented thinking: that is, the use of a sensor mat and a staff-assisted walking routine.

But, as shown earlier, in effect it was the accumulated tension between what was required (care needs) and what was available (care provision) for Mr Harris to walk safely that broke the balancing act of supporting Mr Harris to walk as often as he wanted. In other words, he was stopped from attempting to walk when his difficulty with walking safely outgrew the limited provision of staff assistance. However, instead of providing *more* care in the form of staff assistance to enable Mr Harris to continue to walk, different *forms* of care (within the funding categories of Mobility Care and Fall Prevention) were planned, offering timed and limited staff assistance that could be scheduled. Here we can see an interplay of multiple forces (government funding scheme, financial management of a service provider, and care planning based on medicalized assessments, albeit with embedded economic considerations) and other discourses, such as residents' safety, duty of care for residents and work efficiency. Clearly, the discourse of risk plays a pivotal role in any reconfiguration of care assemblages, while other considerations are hidden in the construction of care plans and the daily routines of care.

From the perspective of care management, a staff-assisted walking routine is an example of providing, as a senior staff member said, the 'best possible care'. Routines were seen by staff as a way to manage unexpected and unpredictable events by organizing residents' movements, in the interests of safety as well as the smooth operation of care work. Despite its restrictions, according to carers, the staff-assisted walking routine had been 'working all right' in assisting Mr Harris with his need to mobilize safely without straining the constraints of funding and staffing levels.

If we return to the notion of a 'right assemblage of care', however, we remember that an assemblage of care only becomes right when it is productive, responsive and supportive – when it enables residents to move, to extend and connect so that they can have a sense of home in the nursing home. Looking at staff-assisted walking routines through the lens of a right assemblage of care, the assemblage did not 'work all right', as staff claimed, because it was designed to be less productive and even to restrict residents from moving at will and from feeling a sense of rightness through being able to connect with people and things outside their rooms. After hours and hours of walking with his wheelie walker, Mr Harris had become inseparable from it. Through walking, his feet were grounded, and his legs became flexible, and that only happened with the aid of his walker. Mr Harris' walker was therefore an indispensable material thing in his assemblage of care to sensorially extend his body to connect with others. His walking habit was badly ruptured when his walker was taken away and those connections were severed. Now he was left sitting in a chair like a statue or a piece of furniture. A staff-assisted walking routine, operating to a fixed procedure or plan, could actually destroy his ability to live beyond his impairments. The once-smooth flow of his movements became blocked and broken. The assemblage of care described in Chapter 3 will not be 'all right' if Mr Harris is left sitting in a chair for long hours before and after a routine walk, without engaging in other activities. Mr Harris's new fall prevention care plan, with its sensor mat alarm and a comfortable chair as its key components, is an assemblage of care that foregrounds safety rather than movement, and supervision rather than assistance. It is an assemblage *not* to enable Mr Harris to walk, but to stop him from walking.

Seen through the lens of assemblages of care, the nature of caring can be revealed as multiplicities; various components of care practices and discourses are assembled and enacted differently in changing circumstances. Some are productive and responsive to residents' efforts to move, while others are less productive or even restrictive, preventing movement and limiting residents' sense of rightness of being-in-the-world-with-others. In the next section, we will further explore the restrictive policies and practices of restraint, their impact on residents' moving or not moving and how that relates to their sense of home in the nursing home.

## Restraint: A Duty of Care?

This section will demonstrate that institutional responses towards residents' attempts to move are heavily mediated by a range of factors: dominant medical discourse of risk and agitation, policies on fall prevention and behavioural management that aim to keep residents safe, and overarching organizing structures that prioritize economic efficiency. Fall prevention measures, such as soft carpet in corridors, non-slip floor coverings and recommended footwear for residents, are practical initiatives that are not really restrictive to residents' movement. However, more restrictive practices do exist in nursing homes. Restraint in the context of aged care facilities is defined in Australian aged care policy as 'any aversive practice, device or action that interferes with any person's ability to make a decision or which restricts their free movement' (Department of Health and Ageing 2012a: 1). The intentional restriction of a resident's voluntary movement or behaviour by the use of a device, or removal of mobility aids, or physical force for behavioural purposes is considered as physical restraint (Department of Health and Ageing 2012a: 24).

Aside from physical restraints, chemical restraints are also used in nursing homes. Chemical restraint refers to the intentional use of medicines that sedate or tranquillize, to control a resident's behaviour when the behaviour to be affected by the active ingredient does not appear to have a medical cause (Department of Health and Ageing 2012a: 25). In nursing homes, if problematic behaviours are interpreted as symptoms of dementia, those behaviours are not considered to be medically 'treatable' conditions. A chemical restraint is thus the use of any drug for disciplinary purposes or staff convenience, rather than having clinical benefits for patients. Pharmacological agents used for restraint, such as antipsychotic or neuroleptic medication, can clearly impair residents' efforts to move. At the time I carried out my fieldwork, the over-medicalization of residents and use of restraint practices gained widespread media attention after an investigation into the death of Bob Spriggs, a former resident at the Older Persons Mental Health Facility at Oakden, in Adelaide, South Australia.

The use of restraint in nursing homes and hospitals often reflects the limited capacity of institutions to care for residents with complex needs due to dementia. This was the case with Mrs Wilson, a resident with late-stage Alzheimer's disease, who was utterly mute. Described by staff as 'a big wanderer', when she was still able to walk, her balance became affected as her dementia progressed. After she had multiple successive falls and badly bruised herself, she was assigned a princess chair in the lounge area. In the case of Mrs Wilson, a princess chair was not intended to be a method of restraint, but it effectively limited her movements even though she was not tied to the chair. While in this chair she would become restless and shuffle her feet. Staff documented these movements as a 'behavioural problem' and described how she often became 'agitated, fought with staff and lashed out from fatigue, pain and confusion'. During a hospital stay, when she was treated for a urinary infection, Mrs Wilson was diagnosed as having 'agitation', and after returning to the nursing home, antipsychotic treatment was added to her medications. As a side effect of this neuroleptic medication, Mrs Wilson became sedated and then her eating and drinking rapidly decreased because she was often drowsy. She eventually returned to hospital with acute kidney injury from severe dehydration and aspiration pneumonia.

As well as from restraint, prolonged sitting could also bring an end to residents' walking. Mr Harris stopped trying to move after becoming exhausted from his attempts to stand up and walk. Staff then said that Mr Harris developed a condition of 'apathy' due to the progression of his Parkinson's disease and that he appeared to be unaffected by and uninterested in his surroundings. In staff readings, his apathetic state was understood as the sole outcome of disease progression. I take a different point of view. I approach this lack of engagement as intimately entwined with the practice of restraint and his receiving very little encouragement to move and to walk. The body becomes unproductive when one's desire to move is no longer assisted and supported, and it begins to atrophy. The problem might appear to be apathy but is really the progressive eradication of all movements, a lack of sensory articulation with other people and things. When right assemblages of care fall apart, one's very desire to move and to stay in touch with the world fades away and eventually vacates the body.

As I observed, residents' movements, if appearing unsafe, would quickly attract staff attention and spontaneous assistance, especially from newly recruited carers or students on work placement. In talking with Mr Dixon, carers tacitly acknowledged that he was trying to get out of his chair in order to walk, a practice that was judged to be unsafe. 'You can feel it. All he (Mr Dixon) wants is to stand up and go. But he could fall at any minute,' they would say. However, instead of joining forces and assisting him to walk, staff mostly urged Mr Dixon to sit back in his chair. 'It's better for Mr Dixon to stay seated,' one worker said. You may ask how staff could think like that. If you could feel his urge to walk, how could stopping Mr Dixon from walking be better for Mr Dixon than assisting him to walk? 'Mr Dixon has a high risk of falls. It's safer for him to remain seated' was the usual response. Clearly, carers' response towards residents' attempts to move is heavily mediated by institutional interpretations of resident movement, which, as we have seen, are largely influenced by the discourse of risk. Risk is a key component of care needs assessment, care planning and care management. I contend, however, that in the nursing home, risk is misconceptualized. Risk did not arise from lack of staff attention and assistance but from residents' efforts to move, and that risk was managed not by providing assistance to residents who desired to move but by physically forcing residents to remain seated.

When residents' attempts to move are persistent, this can further be labelled as 'agitative behaviour' – a behavioural and psychological symptom of dementia. Agitation is seen as causing trouble for family members, caregivers and other service users because while unattended, patients with agitative behaviours may make unsafe movements and injure themselves or others. As we have seen, the medical discourse of agitation is dominant in nursing home settings, as exemplified in the case of Mrs Wilson, who, when confined to her chair, was described as 'restless' and 'senseless'. The Oakden Review report also revealed that residents' movements while seated in chairs were most likely to be perceived by staff as 'pathetic, irrational and harmful' to themselves and others, and thus regarded as 'agitated behaviour', associated with 'restless sleep patterns and episodes of hyperactivity' (Groves et al. 2017: 106). The medical discourse of agitation as a symptom of dementia measures people and their movements against 'the statistically normal, relegating everything that falls beyond this range to the register of the "pathological"' (Smith 2018: 107). The term 'agitation' conjures up the repetitiveness and persistence of residents' attempts to move. These persistent yet failed attempts display certain embodied tensions and reflect both an innermost drive to move and the difficulty of doing so without proper assistance. I contend that what is conceived as 'trouble' is in effect a disjuncture between the assistance residents need and the support that is made available to them. The discourse of risk and the discourse of agitation can reconfigure existing assemblages of care into new assemblages of knowing and doing. If an attempt to move is considered a sign of agitation, residents with dementia are more likely to be rough-handled by staff, prescribed with antipsychotic medication, or physically restrained in a chair. In this sense, the discourse of agitation is a key component in assemblages of care that use restraint to reduce residents' capacities for movement.

From mobility (capacity to move) to a risk of falls (potentially harmful attempt to move), to the 'agitative behaviour' (harmful movements to self and other people), a resident's attempt to move is constantly codified. This influences carers' interpretations of resident movement and indirectly affects the organization of staff attention and assistance. The twin discourses of risk and agitation translate residents' drive to move into something that is harmful that needs to be prevented. The sad result is that chemical and physical restraints are therefore used with residents to eliminate risk, by stopping them from moving at all. Contrary to staff belief that restraint is a practice of care, restricting residents' movements may in effect constitute a form of violence – creating and reinforcing the forces that inhibit residents from sensory engagements with others and therefore reducing their possibility to ever settle and feel at home in the nursing home.

Preventing residents from harm and having falls is seen as important for resident safety and thus has become a fundamental element of how care is practised. While residents in the later stages of dementia, like Mrs Wilson and Mr Dixon, usually have lost the capacity to care about their own safety while moving, their safety becomes a central concern for carers, management and the facility service provider. During the Royal Commission into Aged Care Quality and Safety, Sydney Hearing from 6–17 May 2019, the Royal Commission heard evidence from Professor Henry Brodaty, who gave an example of how a patient with severe Parkinson's disease and moderate dementia lived in the tension between staying safe and taking the risk to walk. The patient's wife was 'very happy for him to walk and to take that risk because his quality of life is more important than his safety' but realized the nursing home has a duty of care and responsibility for residents' safety. Professor Brodaty referred to this tension as existing 'between cotton wool, safety and autonomy and independence [which is] one of these wicked problems that we have in looking after people in nursing homes'

(Royal Commission into Aged Care Quality and Safety 2019: 1903). Fall Prevention is given greater emphasis in the daily operation and management of care delivery than Mobility Care. Resident safety from falls and fall-related injuries is important: it directly involves the duty of care of the organization as well as each individual employee, in both a legal and moral sense.

It becomes evident in the analyses that it is the perspective of the service providers and carers and their medico-legal duty of care and not the people who are cared for that is embedded in current discourses of risk and agitation. The discourses work together to construct a particular kind of care for residents, producing medicalized responses in the form of interventions to prevent harm and falls by restricting movement, as opposed to providing the sensory benefits made possible through assisting bodies to move. As shown here, care, as it is currently constituted in residential aged care, can reduce possibilities for residents to continue to move.

In his conceptualization of the social ethics of care, Rapport (2018) claims that the elderly may be constrained from exercising their free will while being cared for. If resident movement, such as the persistent walking of Mrs Sage and the attempted standing and walking of Mr Dixon, is to be understood as an essence of autonomy – an exercise of free will in Rapport's sense – the type of fall prevention that this section has discussed could be regarded as an infringement of resident autonomy.

## Creating the 'Right Care'

How can a right assemblage of care be created for residents with impaired mobility and cognition? How can they be assisted to move with ease and feel at home in the nursing home? Learning from my work with residents, I started to see that the creation of a right assemblage of care for residents with impaired mobility and cognition to help them continue to move relies on a better interpretation of resident movement. To achieve this, the established discourses of risk and agitation need to be challenged. I will now return to the examples of Mrs Wilson and Mr Dixon to demonstrate how the different interpretations of resident movement – namely, capacity to move in the case of Mrs Wilson and risk of falls in the case of Mr Dixon – could lead to residents having different assemblages of care: some were 'right' – productive and supportive to residents' efforts to move and to have a sense of being-at-home; some were not so 'right' – less productive or even restrictive to residents' efforts to move. If we start with the right understanding of resident movement, new possibilities of doing care with increased responsiveness and flexibility will emerge.

We can start with the example of Mrs Wilson to demonstrate how a different way of interpreting her movements while seated could lead to the creation of a right assemblage of care to overcome the tension she often displayed between moving and staying still. As I described in the previous section, Mrs Wilson was assigned a princess chair to sit in for long hours after having successive falls. Her habit of moving around in the chair was interpreted as 'agitated behaviour' and was subjected to medical diagnosis and pharmaceutical treatment: chemical restraint that severely restrained her movements and even affected her ability to eat and drink. It was the implementation of a 'no restraints' policy in daily care practices at the nursing home that became an opportunity for innovative ideas and technologies to be considered. This was demonstrated in the everyday life of Mrs Wilson, which was transformed when her attempt to move in her chair and to stand up was recognized and she was supported to move. During a week-long period of hospitalization, her medications were reviewed, and the antipsychotic medication was stopped; she was rehydrated and treated for aspiration pneumonia. When she returned to the care facility, her oral intake significantly improved with the antipsychotic medication stopped. Her Mobility Care Plan was also updated after careful assessment of her remaining capacity to move.

One day, I was surprised to see Mrs Wilson not in her princess chair when I walked past the lounge area. Instead, she was sitting in a high-backed day chair, which looked different from the usual lounge chairs. I later realized that the new chair had two special features. First, the seat width of the chair was narrower than that of the princess chair, which left a one-inch gap between the outermost part of her hip and the arm of the chair. Instead of leaning heavily on one arm of her princess chair, which could lead to her feeling unstable, Mrs Wilson could now sit more in the middle of the chair, with her lower arms resting evenly on both of its arms. Secondly, the seat height could be adjusted so that her feet could firmly touch the floor, with a slightly wider than 90-degree angle formed between her thigh and lower leg. Seeing Mrs Wilson in a more normal-looking chair with her feet on the floor, I felt puzzled. Could Mrs Wilson stand up again now that her feet were on the floor? Sitting down in a corner to observe, I was surprised to see Mrs Wilson put her hands on the arm rests and lean forward to lift her buttocks. She froze in that posture for two seconds and then stood up. She maintained the upright posture for a few seconds, with her hands holding onto the arms of the chair. Then she let go of the armrests, stretched her arms forward, and sat back in the chair. Taking a deep breath, she made another move to stand. After she repeated these movements half a dozen times, she seemed tired from the exertion. She sat for a few minutes, leaning her back against the chair with her arms loosely hanging by her side. Then, she started moving again.

With her feet on the floor and her lower arms supported by the arms of the chair, Mrs Wilson could easily push on the chair's armrests to stand up and bend her knees to sit back safely onto her chair. The change of position came with apparent ease because she was grounded: she had something underneath her feet. Certainly, she looked more stable, secure and calm. When a person does not have a sense of 'grounding' or stability, they might seek sensory feedback by trying to find the floor with their feet, leading to an increased risk of falls. Mrs Wilson would feel the weight of her body through her feet, meaning that pressure was distributed throughout her body. She would not feel the same pressure, pain and discomfort in her buttocks as she did while sitting with her body tipped back, as it was in the princess chair. This change in position evidently changed Mrs Wilson's demeanour. Unlike the person who sat in the princess chair looking anxious and distressed, the new Mrs Wilson in her new chair appeared to be quite relaxed. Her body, chair and the ground beneath her came together in a concerted and successful effort to move – stand up and sit down whenever she felt the inclination.

When she was free to sit and stand, Mrs Wilson's everyday life was transformed – she became more grounded and connected with others due to being in control of her own bodily movements. Moving around made her more visible to others. People coming and going said 'Hello!', and although she remained silent, she was at least visible and more likely to be attended to. Moving, fundamentally, is a way to connect and interact. Her simple repetitive motions to sit/stand made Mrs Wilson a distinctive figure in the dementia care unit. People recognized her presence and existence. Family members, visitors, volunteers and students doing work placement often turned to staff asking: 'Who is the old lady doing sit/stand [exercise] in the lounge?'

'It's Mrs Wilson. She is now doing pretty well, isn't she?' carers would reply, with a hint of pride. When in motion, her facial expressions of frustration and confusion were replaced by one of concentration (while moving) and relaxation (while sitting). It was shown in the daily documentation that Mrs Wilson ate more and slept better after the new arrangement with her chair. This is in line with research findings that physical exercise significantly benefits individuals living with dementia in nursing homes (Brett, Traynor and Stapley 2016).

A purposely designed chair and increased staff attention could benefit Mrs Wilson by enabling her to become at ease with making movements. Like walking, changing position is a kinaesthetic form of activity involving whole body movements, balancing on one's feet, in a coupling of perception and action. Feeling the texture of the carpeted floor is to absorb the haptic sense of pressure from underneath one's feet. Standing up is to notice and respond to the sensory inputs that allow one to balance on one's feet. In the closed loop of sensory incorporation and response initiation (perception coupling with action), one can feel just right in standing up. While moving in, and stretching away from and back into the chair, the body moves of its own accord. Neurons in muscles, joints and tendons respond to sensory inputs from touch and pressure and work with the brain to let a person unconsciously know where the body parts are to produce bodily synthesis (Merleau-Ponty 1962) and coordinate movements. The entire nervous system is responsible for the kinaesthetic sense to monitor the body's own movements. In the concerted moving of the head, trunk, limbs, feet and hands, in relation to the chair and floor, one experiences the particular feeling of energy being exerted. This feeling is accompanied by a sensation of strain and labour from the contracting of muscles. A sense of effort is the conscious awareness of one's own voluntary movements, which is crucial for the judgement of personal actions and is at the core of a sense of self expanding to relate to the external world. Although Mrs Wilson may not have had a conscious awareness of her own efforts, she still lived in and through the preconscious processes of desiring-production and synthesis.

The example of Mrs Wilson demonstrates that, for the elderly people with severe physical and cognitive impairments, the sense of becoming-at-home in the nursing home is deeply rooted in their innermost drive to move, to flow in and out of positions. Residents in the later stages of dementia could temporarily break away from their bodily impairments and feel some control over their movements. Assistance from others can be attracted into their attempted movements so that their various forms of 'becoming-moving' could be reassembled and rearranged into shared efforts. The synthesis of efforts of residents, carers, assistive devices and technologies could thus leverage the tension between moving and staying still.

This account of how Mrs Wilson could continue to move through thoughtful staff attention and a purposely designed chair challenges the biomedical conceptualization of residents' seated movements as 'agitation', which is a behavioural and psychological symptom of dementia. Contrary to the belief that these movements are pathological markers that ought to be controlled and reduced by the application of biomedical and psychosocial interventions, residents' efforts of moving in correspondence with innovative assistive technologies could potentially transform daily care practices and residents' everyday experiences. Supporting residents like Mrs Wilson to continue to move as much as they can and keep attempting to do so is important because, as Rapport (2018) argues in his work on social ethics of care, believing that their autonomy is not violated is central to residents' having a sense of home in the nursing home. Movement is an important way of exercising free will even *outside of* conscious choice and action.

I now want to return to the question that I asked at the beginning of this section – namely, how to create a right assemblage of care for residents with impaired mobility and cognition to move 'all right' and consequently feel at home in the nursing home. As shown in the example of Mrs Wilson, the creation of a right assemblage of care only becomes possible if movement is not misinterpreted as risk or agitation but as the resident's effort to feel 'right', have autonomy and so feel a sense of home. To further illustrate this point, I will now turn to the example of Mr Dixon. Staff misinterpretation of his need to stand and walk could have ultimately led to an assemblage of care that was not right for him. Challenging the misinterpretation meant that innovative ideas and technologies could be integrated into his care organization to make a right assemblage of care for Mr Dixon and residents like him.

This analysis could start by carefully comparing Mr Dixon's particular bodily condition to that of Mrs Wilson and Mr Harris. Each of these residents experienced their movements differently. Bodily impairments governed whether and how those residents could continue to walk. Mr Dixon experienced constant fluctuations of attention, mobility and cognition. He needed staff assistance to walk but only during the moments when he became aware of the world and started his attempts to move. In contrast, Mrs Wilson did not need staff assistance to stand and required little assistance to walk. Other residents could hardly walk without staff assistance; for example, Mr Harris could not initiate movements without staff assistance after his condition deteriorated. Mr Dixon's moments of being able to walk were unpredictable. Staff assistance in response to his attempted movements thus could not be prescheduled in care planning within a fixed temporal structure. In fact, he was likely to become alert and attempt to move at any given moment and to need prompt staff assistance to prevent him from falling. Two aspects therefore became pivotal in assisting Mr Dixon to move safely. First, Mr Dixon needed to be monitored for movements, even while sitting still and asleep, although at these times, staff assistance was not always needed. Second, once Mr Dixon started attempting to walk, he needed to be attended to promptly, and assistance then became essential.

Being prescribed a Fall Prevention Plan with a sensor mat alarm as its key component, Mr Dixon was effectively monitored for potential movements, which covered the first aspect of assisting him to move safely. This ongoing monitoring does not require continuous supervision. A sensor mat is innovative technology that can capture early signs of residents' attempts to move. Staff only need to respond with assistance when the resident starts moving, setting the alarm off. This gives residents a degree of freedom to walk safely, and reassurance to carers, who are less stressed by uncertain or excessive demands for assistance. So the use of a sensor mat alarm may potentially aid in two ways – by protecting residents from falls and improving their mobility, as long as prompt staff assistance is provided to residents whenever they set off the alarm.

Nevertheless, as I discussed in the previous section and also in Chapter 4, Mr Dixon's Fall Prevention Plan, as an assemblage of care, was created to reduce his risk of falls, not for the purpose of assisting him to continue walking as he wished; thus it did not formally include the prescription of staff assistance to help him to continue walking. According to his Fall Prevention Plan, carers were required to 'check on him', not to assist him to walk; in fact, they would usually assist him to sit back into his chair. Assisting Mr Dixon to sit down (rather than to stand and walk) could not be considered as the right care for Mr Dixon, either as planned exercise or simply to follow his expressed wish. Following this chain of analysis, Mr Dixon's Fall Prevention Plan was not a right assemblage of care for him, because his potential for movement was interpreted according to a single key component – the discourse of risk – as unsafe and unnecessary. The corollary to that is that the walking needed to be stopped by sitting him in a chair.

To create a right assemblage of care for Mr Dixon, his movements in the chair needed to be interpreted in terms of his mobility, including his capacity and strength for moving. His seemingly unsafe walking was neither senseless nor meaningless. It should have been interpreted as his longing for sensory extensions and connections, both as an endeavour and as an invitation – an opportunity to grasp supportive other material things and beings, to both assist and enable residents to keep walking. Carers are given training sessions, emanating from the discourse of risk, on how to mitigate the risk of unsafe walking, but they might be better equipped to understand the complexities of this topic if they look beyond the discourse of risk. This may help them to cultivate what Kleinman (2009) calls the 'empathic imagination' and unsettle taken-for-granted notions of the right ways of caring for vulnerable residents.

From a staff perspective, prompt staff assistance in response to the spontaneous movements of residents like Mr Dixon is only made possible within a care management structure that has less emphasis on time management and rigid schedules. As previously discussed in the subsection of 'routines', organizing prompt staff assistance within the constraints of staffing and funding levels is problematic. Institutional routine care practice promotes regularity and encourages efficiency. Within the routinized daily operation of care activities, there is at present little flexibility for the provision of prompt staff assistance. To overcome the tension between a resident's urgent need for assistance and the prompt availability of that assistance, increasing flexibility in care organization and management is crucial.

Meanwhile, assistive technologies and equipment are thought useful when they fit residents' bodies and conditions and as long as they can reduce the use of human labour and improve overall efficiency. As shown in this section, a right assemblage of care for Mrs Wilson to stand and sit safely did not require the element of unscheduled staff assistance. The combination of support from the adjustable chair and the occasional attention of staff members on the floor was sufficient for Mrs Wilson to do stand–sit on her own. Her sit/stand exercise was safe for her to do, as she was unable to actually take steps and walk. After standing for a few seconds, she would sit back into her chair. It is true that the adjustable chair may not have fitted her after she became no longer weight-bearing. But in the knowledge that a right assemblage of care just requires tinkering in order to go on supporting residents' efforts to move, other innovative ideas and technologies could have been integrated into her care as needed.

## Notes

1. Day shifts for care workers included: from 7 AM to 3 PM, 7 AM to 2 PM, 7 AM to 12 PM and 7 AM to 11 AM. The 7 AM to 11 AM shift was a 'floating shift' that could be relocated to other areas whenever the workload in this area was reduced; for example, due to changes in resident numbers.
2. Tubigrip is a specially designed elasticated tubular bandage that provides firm but comfortable support for sprains, strains and weak joints. It can also be used to reduce swelling and to keep dressings in place.
3. According to research that the Australian Nursing and Midwifery Federation (ANMF) commissioned, the current aged care resident in Australia receives roughly 2.5 hours of care per day, and the staffing mix is usually 70% personal care workers (PCWs) and 15% both registered nurses (RNs) and enrolled nurses (ENs). On Wednesday 13 February 2019, the Federal Secretary of ANMF, Annie Butler, appeared before the Royal Commission into Aged Care Quality and Safety and explained why mandated minimum staffing levels and skills mix are an essential part of any solution to ensure safe care for every elderly resident (ANMF 2019). The ANMF's research has shown that an average of 4.3 nursing and care hours are needed each day and they also identified the ideal skills mix required to deliver this care. In order to achieve the recommended care time, the ANMF proposed that by 1 January 2022 average care time should increase to 3.75 hours per day per resident with a minimum of one RN per 30 residents during day shifts and one RN on other shifts, and by 1 January 2025, average care time provided to residents should increase to a minimum of 4.3 hours, with a minimum of one RN per 15 residents during day shifts and one RN per 30 residents during evening and night shifts (Cheu 2018).

# 6 CARING AT THE THRESHOLD OF LIFE AND DEATH

## Eating and Not Eating at the End of Life

In his Afterword to the articles collected in *The Australian Journal of Anthropology* special issue 'Moralities of Care in Later Life', Rapport (2018) cites Patricia Gillespie's account of her mother's refusal of medications and food for several weeks prior to her death. Rapport uses this example to suggest that caring should not infringe upon the autonomy of the elderly at the end of their lives. He asserts, 'Over and against an impersonal, social-structural or institutional power is an existential power', the human capacity to 'have scant respect for the rules', as reflected in Patricia Gillespie's mother's decision '… to set and pursue an individual path for oneself' (Rapport 2018: 251). Rapport represents the elderly person's starving to death as a deliberate choice and an agentic action – the expression of one's free will to shape one's own course of life and death.

In examining the relations between food, agency and care for older people who are at the end of their lives, Rapport shows how eating and not eating are centrally placed at this critical life course juncture. If one stops eating, it leads to malnutrition and, eventually, death. The regular incorporation of food into self is essential to physical survival. To eat or not eat is thus not simply an individual choice over food; it can be an individual choice between life and death. For Rapport, it is possible for a frail elderly person to take control over their own life and death through taking control of their eating, and that choice should be respected and supported by the people around them. As starving to death voluntarily indicates a wish to die, Rapport suggests that Patricia Gillespie's mother was executing full control over her own life and death through her deliberate choice to reject food. To eat to live or not eat to die is about acting according to one's own will, free from the influence of external forces. In the context of allowing frail elderly people to starve to death, Rapport defines ethical care as 'a particular kind of social framework or environment that endeavours to give an appropriate proportionality to autonomy and inclusion' (2018: 250). Within that framework, individual autonomy is experienced as maintaining one's 'abiding authorship of his or her life-project(s) but also authority, determining the course of that life and the trajectory of its becoming' (2018: 255). With use of the word 'proportionality', Rapport is proposing a version of ethical care that is balanced 'between engagement and inclusion on the one hand, and a preservation of autonomy and personal sovereignty on the other; between action and inaction' (2018: 250). Here, Rapport is referring to those impersonal powers that inhibit or prevent the elderly from exercising free will. His emphasis on the overarching importance of autonomy in ethical care is well considered. We saw in Chapter 5 how restrictive practices were placed on nursing home residents, practices that prevented them from either walking or standing. In effect, this blocked the flow of their 'productive desire' to keep moving and hence all the benefits to mental and physical health that we know movement brings. Although for residents with cognitive changes a productive desire could no longer manifest itself in a conscious exercise of free will, the detrimental effects of inhibitive, restrictive forces on them can still be profound.

In this chapter, I turn to the lives of nursing home residents with dementia to explore the vexed question of eating and not eating as it applies to frail elderly people during the very last stages of their lives. For the residents I observed, not eating was marked by ambiguity and ambivalence. Staff and family did not unanimously agree that residents could self-determine to not eat, and thus die. Unlike Patricia Gillespie's mother, who had insight into how the regular consumption of food is essential to physical survival, many elderly people in residential care do not have this insight due to severe cognitive impairments related to late-stage dementia. In other words, they would not be able to make a choice over life or death by taking control of their eating. They cannot make a considered choice and take a deliberate action to stop eating. In short, for nursing home residents with severe cognitive impairments, eating and not eating is not about taking control, be it over food or the timing of life and death.

In questioning Rapport's position that not eating is always an individual choice, this chapter critically examines eating and not eating through the lens of productive desire (Deleuze and Guattari 1977). One's appetite to ingest food is really a powerful desire to attract and incorporate food, to fill and to nourish the body. A lack of appetite indicates a weakening of the productive forces that impel one to eat. In the field, I observed how appetites appeared to be triggered by a home-cooked dish, a companion, or a gentle stroke on the throat, or diminished by texture-modified food and fluids as well as insufficient staff assistance.

At the very last stages of their lives, residents' relationship with food is often complicated by severe cognitive impairments, physical eating difficulties, medications as well as assistive technologies and policies that shape the daily practices of nutrition care. Sensory and perceptual changes may lead to reduced appetite. Chewing and swallowing problems due to muscle paralysis can be a choking risk. The use of sedative medication may hasten that decline to a tipping point, where, in compliance to policy, residents are prescribed texture-modified food and fluids to which they close their mouths and stop eating. Using the example of Mrs Brie in this chapter, I want to explore how residents become moved or impelled to eat or not eat according to the vicissitudes of their productive desire. Mapping the flows of their movements and marking the tipping points and thresholds of forces that are productive or counterproductive will allow me to reveal the complex entanglement of (mal)nourished bodies, sensorily-modified food and fluids, (in)attentive practices of feeding residents, and the challenge of caring for deteriorating and dying bodies.

Feeling accompanied, comforted and at ease is at the heart of people feeling at home in residential care. For residents to feel at home in care during that final process of their lives, a right care must always be responsive to their desires, even as appetites wax and wane. For example, I observed how Mrs Brie could still enjoy eating when it gave her a taste of home, as described in the next section.

## Taste of Home

In the last stage of Alzheimer's disease, almost all the cognitive functions of Mrs Brie were severely impaired. She could no longer walk or talk. Sitting in her princess chair parked in the lounge, she was often seen snoozing on and off or staring into the distance with no facial expression. Yet, lunchtime (see Illustration 6.1) was the highlight of the day for Mrs Brie, as Heather, her eldest daughter, often came in then for a visit.

When she heard Heather's voice greeting staff, Mrs Brie would start moving in her chair and look around. Her face lit up with a soft glow when she saw Heather. While on any day, she may or may not have recognized Heather, she still looked eager to have her company. Shared between mother and daughter was a love for food and cooking. On each of her visits, Heather brought a home-cooked meal: one day it might be a tomato-cheese quiche, on another a roast beef and rocket leaf sandwich, thoughtfully prepared with the sandwich crusts cut off. Over a slice of her mother's favourite – home-baked apple pie – Heather chatted about her siblings, relatives, friends, children and grandchildren. Although Mrs Brie showed little expression as Heather talked, she was usually interested in the food on her plate. Having lunch with Heather became a regular and pleasurable social event for Mrs Brie; the company of Heather and the home-cooked

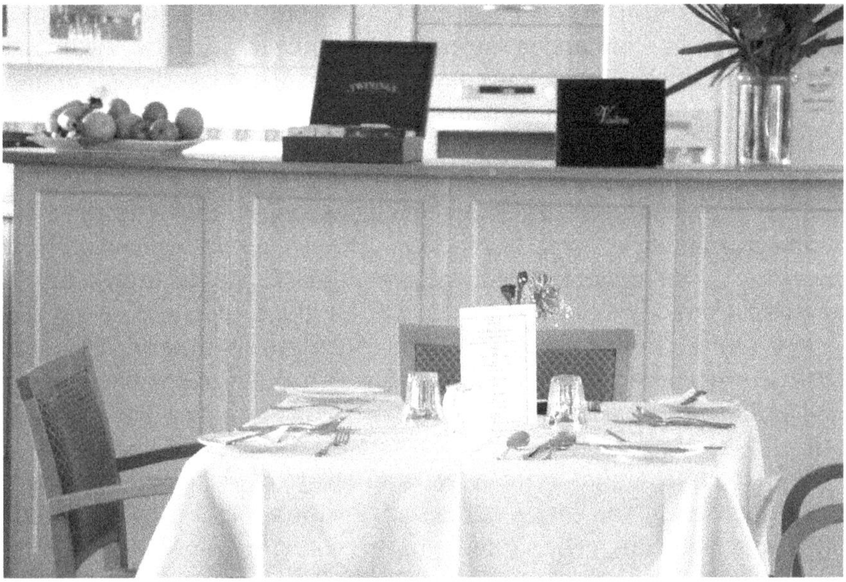

ILLUSTRATION 6.1. Dining area. Image provided courtesy of Helpinghand.

meal was something to anticipate and to enjoy. The senses and sensibilities associated with food and eating cannot be reduced to simple nutrition or physical survival. Eating is intimately entangled with relationships; in this case, the intimacy between mother and daughter and their connection through food. Similarly, the significance of family visitors bringing a favourite food to their institutionalized relatives has often been discussed in other nursing home research around the world (High and Rowles 1995; Rowles and High 2003).

As she ate, Mrs Brie often used her fingers to pick up a small portion from the plate and put it into her mouth. She could not handle normal cutlery due to her arthritic fingers. Eating with her fingers was the way Mrs Brie engaged with her food. Connecting with her meal by touching, holding, watching and tasting, she exhibited a range of facial expressions, showing interest, contentment, pleasure or surprise. Eating with her fingers allowed Mrs Brie to cultivate nourishing connections with her food beyond its purely nutritional value.

Bodily movements involved in eating and drinking are an essential part of the lived reality of human lives: '... from the very beginning, we all have mouths that open and close, and that edibles and other things are and can be put inside them' (Sheets-Johnstone 2011: 122). Nevertheless, consuming food is never as simple as the opening and closing of the mouth, especially during the later stages of life. In his nursing home study on food,

Savishinsky (2003) cites the classic study of physician Walter Cannon, which found that human food intake can be motivated both by nutritional need and a desire for certain sensations of delight. In the latter case, Cannon said, the person 'seeks satisfaction, not relief' (1939: 75 as in Savishinsky 2003: 116). Clearly, food is both nutrition and pleasure. Eating is often thought of as involving a hunger pang (a sense of needing and wanting) and an appetite (a sense of craving and liking tastes), both leading to the actual consuming of food. Leon Kass, a physician and biochemist, also suggests, '... the germ of appetite governs, guides, and integrates awareness and action: Appetite or desire, not DNA, is the deepest principle of life' (1994: 48). According to Fox, '... our appetites and our desires play a part in structuring our waking lives ... these desires not only affect our thoughts and feelings, but also how we are motivated to act on a daily basis' (2012: 106).

The type of food that one consumes also plays a role in one's eating or not eating. Seeing, smelling, touching and tasting something good is stimulating and motivating. The various sensory properties of food, including its taste, aroma, temperature and texture, actually trigger the act of swallowing (Loret 2015). The actual or imagined presence of food may also trigger a strong desire to eat. Carers I worked with noted that triggers as simple as seeing someone eat can encourage residents to eat something themselves. Handling food with one's fingers, as Mrs Brie seemed to enjoy doing, can also act as a trigger through sensory stimulation, which is helpful in releasing digestive juices and enzymes. The nerve endings on fingertips can relay the message that one is about to eat, thereby preparing the stomach for digestion.

Alongside the body and the food itself, there were also other material things and persons involved in residents' eating. Modified eating and drinking utensils, such as a lipped (high-sided) plate, adapted cutlery and a non-spill cup, are often used in aged care facilities to enable residents like Mrs Brie to continue feeding themselves. Sitting with her mother, Heather closely watched how Mrs Brie took food from the plate to her mouth or drank from the feeding cup with its vented lid and drinking spout, and from time to time she carefully guided her mother's hand to her mouth. Mrs Brie would have been unable to drink without the assistance of Heather and the purposely designed feeder cup.

The hands (of Mrs Brie and Heather), the feeder cup, the mouth and the food were drawn together and assembled into a productive process in which the body first desired and was then moved to eat. Food is not just a passive object that is consumed. Its presence may trigger movements, so that the hands, lips, teeth, tongue and cheeks entwine in the event of eating. A mouth opens to the feeder cup because a desire to incorporate what is contained within makes the mouth move. A tongue starts the processes of chewing, grinding and salivating when the touch of food on its tip signals the form and texture of the edible in one's mouth. In this sense, food and fluids can be thought of, using the term 'desiring-machine' of Deleuze and Guattari (1977), as food-machine and fluids-machine, producing a pattern of affects and motions. A set of dentures and a piece of buttered bread or a plate of noodle soup, a spoon with a rubber handle and a shaking hand due to Parkinson's disease all synchronize to produce the event of eating. In holding a small portion of apple pie, which had a taste of her previous life, the arthritic fingers of Mrs Brie entered into relation with the food in a way that allowed those fingers to do what they otherwise could not do. This assemblage opened up new connections and possibilities to re-create a familiar sense of home.

In that light, we should start to understand aged residents' eating as an event, or process of desiring-production. In moving food and fluids into and through the body, the hands (of Mrs Brie and Heather), the tongue, the feeder cup and the tea all worked in coordination and synchronization to produce movements of desire. For Mrs Brie, eating was productive: the possibility of Mrs Brie feeding herself with ease and enjoyment was actualized through a right assemblage of care, despite her condition, where arthritic fingers and confusion from Alzheimer's disease rendered eating a challenging task for her.

In nursing homes, attempts are made to cater to residents' likes, dislikes and preferences, which is in line with the research finding that staff could combine 'a medical attitude towards food (appreciating it for its nutritional value) with a caring attitude (which tries to accommodate and please a person)' (Harbers, Mol and Stollmeyer 2002: 216). When care facilities lay emphasis on both the quantity and the quality of food, eating and drinking not only play a pivotal role in terms of residents' nutrition and hydration but also increasingly become events of pleasure and enjoyment (see Illustration 6.2). Residents' eating is considered to be not only need- but also desire-driven. Cooking, and eating afterwards, is regularly organized in the facilities as a type of lifestyle activity for residents who do not have eating difficulties. How the sight and taste of a birthday cake, the smell and sound of a BBQ, and the touch and flavour of freshly baked goods could cheer residents up and put a smile on their faces helped me to 'appreciate the many pleasures the senses stimulate in the elderly and how many meanings food may carry for them' (Savishinsky 2003: 117).

The example of Mrs Brie feeding herself demonstrates that the assemblage of a favourite home-cooked dish, the company of Heather, and eating with fingers and modified utensils could jointly contribute to Mrs Brie's feeling of being-at-home in the nursing home. Yet, the severe deteriorations of

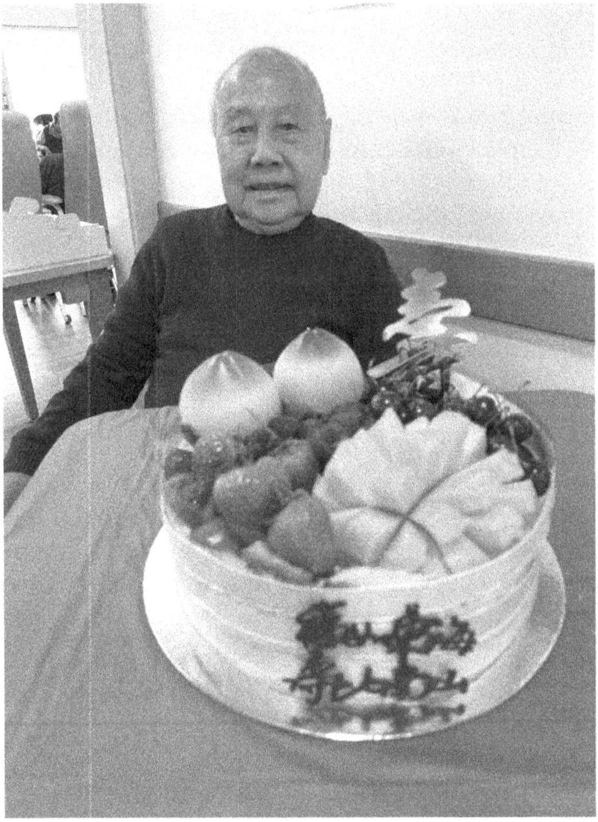

**ILLUSTRATION 6.2.** A resident posing with his birthday cake decorated using the Chinese character 'longevity'. Image provided courtesy of Elder Chinese Home.

the last stages of life often mean that residents are living in a kind of tension between eating and not eating. Let's view eating not as a simple binary of eating and not eating but as a rhizomatic becoming, in order to trace the multiple and at times contested threads as they meet, entangle or break apart. If residents' moving and not moving are thought of as becomings, as illustrated often throughout this book, there are some points where the event of eating becomes ruptured – where residents lose interest and stop eating. These ruptures are related to their difficulties with ingesting food due to medication or a medical condition such as late-stage dementia. In the next section, I want to describe how a period of hospitalization and use of sedative medication can lead to a 'tipping point' where residents like Mrs Brie are no longer able to consume the food they once enjoyed, food that made eating and living pleasurable.

## Fed with 'Mash and Jelly'

Mrs Brie experienced a tipping point in her eating when she had a urinary infection and was sent to hospital. A dramatic change in carers and environment, and the interruption of her lunch routine with Heather, left her severely disoriented. She fought with hospital staff during care routines and was diagnosed with 'agitation'. She was prescribed antipsychotic medication during her hospital stay. Due to a lack of improvement, antipsychotic medication was also added to her medications after her return to the nursing home. In a similar situation as that for residents like Mrs Wilson, described in Chapter 5, Mrs Brie's food consumption rapidly decreased due to the side effects of the antipsychotic medication. She ate little, as she was often drowsy under the influence of the sedative. After several near misses of choking, Mrs Brie was reassessed by the speech pathologist as having dysphagia (swallowing difficulty) and needing a vitaminized diet and thickened fluids. Like many residents with chewing and swallowing problems, Mrs Brie started having 'mash and jelly', texture-modified food and fluids.

In nursing homes, texture modification of food and fluid is regarded as a dysphagia management measure to support certain residents with eating and drinking. Texture modification changes solid food, making it chopped, minced or liquidized to ease residents' difficulty with moving food into the body. When solid food is not completely broken down through chewing, it poses a choking risk to residents. Choking occurs when the trachea is completely or partially blocked by food, liquid or another object, obstructing airflow (Queensland Department of Health 2019). It has been identified as the second most common cause of preventable death in residential aged care (Ibrahim et al. 2017). As a solution to this choking risk, texture-modified food is then prescribed to make the process of eating safer and easier for residents like Mrs Brie. As staff informed me, 'All she needs to do is to open her mouth to eat and close her mouth to swallow'.

Food is texture-modified in the interests of care: assisting with residents' chewing and swallowing and offering protection from choking. In the context of care, not only the provision of food but also what food is provided is a practice of care. However, the question of whether modified food encourages residents with decreased appetite to eat is debatable. For people eating a normal diet, food texture is an important indicator of what is being consumed. Through the mechanical papillae formed on the surface of the tongue, people can feel the form and texture and recognize the food through chewing in between the teeth. Texture modification can take away those sensory properties: the food will be less tasty and harder to recognize. Mrs Brie was observed to move food around in her mouth with an expression of bafflement. In effect, I also had trouble recognizing what was served to Mrs Brie, either by visual examination, smelling or tasting: it looked like a plate with three scoops of white, green and brown 'mash', which was tasteless.

The pleasurable sensations of eating, provided by the senses of sight, smell, taste and touch, are largely felt when we make the subtle tongue and cheeks movements involved in chewing and swallowing. Making efforts to chew, breaking down solid food through the tongue movements of extending, contracting, raising and lowering is important not only to process solid food but also to release saliva and instigate the act of swallowing. When Mrs Brie was stopped from making her own effort of chewing and then swallowing, she could make little sense any more of her eating.

Unlike home-cooked and often strongly flavoured dishes, texture-modified food is usually bland and smooth; it produces few sensations, even though it is easier to swallow. If we look at eating through the lens of Deleuze's concept of multiplicity, with diminished sensory elements (e.g. the shape and colour of food), decreased intensities (e.g. blandness) and reduced dimensions (e.g. the absence of chewing), the nature of eating, as desiring-production, connection, activity and enjoyment, is completely changed. Being fed now with mash, Mrs Brie lost something profoundly productive and connective that previously had allowed her to experience all that her mouth and arthritic fingers could jointly perform. With movements of desire so restricted by the modified food, there is hardly any productive desire left to impel a mouth to open and to eat. Despite the good intention of a dysphagia management plan, the eating of Mrs Brie further deteriorated after she was served pureed meals. She turned her head away from the spoon proffered by staff and firmly closed her mouth. Instead of assisting her to eat better and more safely, food had become an object of aversion.

A similar example relates to fluids. When ordinary drinking water, a daily necessity to health and physical survival, is texture-modified to reduce choking risk, it becomes an object of distaste. On one occasion, I was stopped by a resident in the dining area asking for 'a glass of real water'. He pointed to a plastic cup half-filled with a jelly-like, orange-coloured fluid and said, 'This is not real water. It's yuck. I want real water.' With nods of his head, he emphasized the word 'real' several times. So as not to disappoint him, I went to a staff member with his request. I was told the resisdent was not permitted to have unthickened clear water due to his high choking risk. Curious as to why the elderly man would long for a sip of clear water, I went to a staff member and asked for a taste of what he is usually given. He was absolutely right. Thickened fluid is NOT real water. I had an unpleasant sensation in my mouth after having only a half-mouthful of the 'jelly' – this was indeed nothing like normal drinking water.

Health researchers have noted that for residents in the later stages of dementia who cannot express their needs and preferences, staff consideration of residents' food choices and individual preferences reach a certain 'tipping point' and then stop (Milte et al. 2017). In its submission to the Royal Commission into Aged Care Quality and Safety, the Dietitians Association of Australia (2019: 15) draws on its members' observations to conclude that residents have extremely limited choices with modified texture diets, with some facilities only offering three vegetable options: mashed potatoes, mashed pumpkin or mashed carrots. The lack of enjoyable nutritious food and limited food and fluid choices is highly consequential for residents with chewing and swallowing difficulties: they close their mouths to food and stop eating. This happens when eating is no longer pleasurable and becomes disconnected from any feelings of being at ease and comforted. Residents closing their mouths to food leads to a further challenge to care practices. In the next section, I will explore this phenomenon and its multiple meanings and implications.

## Closing One's Mouth to Food: Caring with Ambiguity and Ambivalence

In nursing homes, the phenomenon of residents closing their mouths to food is understood in a number of different ways. Residents' refusal of food may be considered, as in the case of Patricia Gillespie's mother, as purposeful, as a self-determined wish to die. Reporting from his North American nursing home study, Savishinsky (2003) described how staff attitudes towards residents' decisions to starve to death were divided. Some staff were sympathetic with residents' wish to die and stopped encouraging them to eat, while others disapproved of their colleagues' support for what they saw as assisted suicide. In the Australian nursing homes where I did my fieldwork, such a wish is respected at the facility level and supported with planned care. For example, a female resident was not pressed to eat, and her care plan was carefully adjusted to maintain hydration and comfort after she, with support from her family, clearly expressed her wish to stop eating and to die. For residents with full cognitive capacities, their decision to stop eating is considered as their chosen way to end their life.

Closing the mouth to food could also, however, be seen as residents protesting against how they are fed. When they lose capacity to handle cutlery, residents are usually assisted by staff with the process of taking food from the plate to the mouth. For these residents, as staff said, eating is no longer feeding oneself but is a process of being fed by others. The involvement of staff in the taking in of each mouthful of food profoundly changes how eating is experienced. Once, I saw a care worker blending vitaminized meat and vegetable together with added milk and putting the liquidized mixture into a feeder cup for a resident. 'She only takes a tiny bit each time if I feed her using a teaspoon. Instead, a drink will be a lot easier and faster,' she said. Care staff were often too busy to take more than five minutes to feed one resident because they had other residents who also needed help. Spending longer time with one resident meant that other residents needed to wait, and their food would be cold by the time it was their turn. Sadly, what was considered as a quick fix by the carer gave a bad taste to the resident: after a small sip, the old woman had a bewildered expression on her face. She firmly pressed her lips together when she was urged to have another sip of the 'drink'.

Staff involvement in residents' eating can also change how residents' experiences of eating could be understood, communicated and considered. This is especially so in the situation where residents with advanced dementia are being assisted to eat. Taking full responsibility for resident safety from choking and burns, staff often rely on their own experience and judgement when feeding residents with dementia. Once, when Maureen was feeding Mrs Anderson, a resident in late-stage Alzheimer's disease, Mrs Anderson made a clear utterance, loud enough for Maureen and me to hear. 'It's hot', she said. Maureen was alarmed and stopped feeding with an expression of disbelief. With her left index finger she touched the pureed beef on the spoon. 'I'm sure it's not hot. I left the lid open for quite a while before I started,' Maureen said. She double-checked to ensure that Mrs Anderson's food was not too hot. She changed to another spoon and continued to feed Mrs Anderson. 'It's hot.' Mrs Anderson said again. She looked into the distance in front of her and swallowed without much expression. By this time, I was convinced that Mrs Anderson was not complaining about her food being too hot. 'It's great that Mrs Anderson is talking again. Is that because you are here watching her eating?' Maureen said jokingly. This scenario suggested that while the utterances of residents with advanced dementia were not completely ignored, neither were they taken as accurate accounts of their experiences. Staff mostly relied on their own experience for clinical judgement when feeding residents.

Residents are not only *how* they eat but also *what* they eat. Mrs Brie was classified as a 'soft diet' and requiring supervision when she could feed herself; after her nutrition care plan was updated, she was in the 'vitaminized diet' category, needing full staff assistance. As described by Laird (1979) forty years ago in American nursing homes, eating can come to define residents as those who can walk to the dining room for meals, and those grouped as 'feeders', who have to be hand-fed in their rooms. Residents' experiences of eating and drinking are inevitably shaped by the sort of assistance that is made available in an institutional setting. Residents have less control over what and how to eat while being fed. But they do retain control over a key movement involved in eating: the opening and closing of the mouth. While the opening of the mouth initiates the eating process, closing will stop it. Oral feeding becomes impossible when residents close their mouths to food. In his ethnography, Savishinsky reports that residents closing their mouths when being fed was considered their 'rejection of food', which 'may constitute a resident's reappropriation of their body from those who clean, dress, fill and empty it' (2003: 119).[1] Clearly, in nursing homes, residents' rejection of food can bring to the fore multiple and complex (mis)understandings about physical survival and social relations.

When residents stop eating, are in the later stages of dementia, and are unable to verbally express their needs, likes and dislikes, closing the mouth to food can become a site of contested meaning. In my observations, I found that families of residents were inclined to interpret this as a non-verbal expression of their dislike for the food, and they would regularly advocate for their loved ones and attempt to negotiate with staff for alternatives. While some staff sympathized, others upheld a medical opinion that residents closing their mouth to food, or holding onto food in their mouth, is a swallowing problem, therefore reflecting neither like nor dislike. They reasoned that residents had a reduced appetite and hence a decreased desire for food. Accordingly, they interpreted residents' refusal to eat food as indicative of an absence of the need for nutrition: 'Do they need so much food while sitting all day doing nothing?' nurses and carers would often say. A resident turning their head away from food was also interpreted by nursing staff as a sign that they had lost interest in eating, an indicator of 'withdrawal behaviour', characteristic of the medicalized condition of 'apathy'.

Not eating, then, is a condition with multiple ambiguous meanings; however, what matters in nursing homes is the ambivalence I saw around the question of how to care for these not-eating residents. When eating solid food is no longer permitted or pleasurable for fear of choking, and not eating is easier for the body but life-threatening, finding a right way to care is vital. One day at lunchtime in the dining area, I observed how, despite his persistent attempts, Mike, a registered nurse working in the dementia unit, could not feed Mrs Brie with her lunch, as she firmly closed her mouth to the spoon he offered. Looking worried, Mike said, 'Mrs Brie didn't eat this morning and for the whole of yesterday. She's only had a milkshake. She can't last living on milkshakes.' Not eating, we know, can have dire consequences. Unable to access food by themselves, residents with advanced dementia will starve if they do not consume the food delivered by carers on a spoon. Residents who stop eating will eventually become malnourished and die.

Some staff in the nursing homes expressed their opinion that difficulties with swallowing and eating are due to the progression of their medical condition. This view maintains that, as dementia is irreversible, residents in later stages of dementia, like Mrs Brie, will inevitably stop eating due to the progression of their condition, which marks the imminence of death. During the dying process, the need for fluid and food reduces and is eventually totally eliminated. As not eating is part of dying, there is no need for intervention if residents close their mouths to food during the very last stages of their lives. Forcing a dying person to eat can cause choking. Or it can cause aspiration, which happens when the person 'inhales' food or fluid into the lungs and which can be painful, or even fatal.

However, the issue is not that simple. The starving to death of residents with advanced dementia may also be the consequence of neglect and abuse. In that case it is premature death due to malnutrition, which needs to be addressed. In residential aged care in Australia, studies have identified a prevalence of malnutrition from 22% up to 50% (Dietitians Association of Australia 2019: 8). In an Australian survey representing 64,256 residential beds, over the 2015 and 2016 financial years, the average total spend on the raw food and ingredients budget alone was $6.08 per aged care resident per day (Hugo et al. 2018). Calling malnutrition the 'silent faceless abuser', experts warn that malnourished residents are 'starving to death' (Neil 2019).

In contrast to Patricia Gillespie's mother, who had clearly articulated her wish to starve to death, Mrs Brie might not have been making a deliberate choice to die. As Chapter 2 illustrated, using the example of Mrs Sage, making a wish or will in the mind becomes unlikely, if not utterly impossible, for residents in later stages of dementia. Unlike residents who can still make their own decision to stop eating, either because they wish to die or as a protest against the food and how it is served, residents in later stages of dementia are hardly taking deliberate actions or making informed choices when they close their mouths to food. They would barely comprehend the correlations between opening the mouth, ingesting food and their physical survival. In other words, they do not eat to live or reject food to die.

Like Mrs Wilson, Mrs Brie was affected by antipsychotic medication and was tipped over the edge of functioning with her limited remaining capacity. Closing her mouth to food was surely related to the change of diet from soft to vitaminized, prescribed as an intervention to her swallowing difficulty and choking risk. She might have refused to eat because she disliked a mash or jelly that tasted awful. She might have lost interest in eating when it produced more discomfort than pleasure. She might have lost any remnant of her innermost drive to move or eat due to the sedating medication she was given.

Knowing that life is approaching its end for these very frail nursing home residents who close their mouths to food, some staff members and families do not work strictly to the prescriptive rules. Instead, they acknowledge the ambiguity and ambivalence that is involved in humane caring for these most vulnerable elderly people at the very last stages of their lives. According to Musolino and her colleagues, this pairing of ambiguity and ambivalence lies at the heart of desire (Musolino, Warin and Gilchrist 2018: 546). In their study on young women's eating disorders, the authors use Bauman (1991) to argue that 'ambiguity constructs knowledge that designates opposing states, and ambivalence directs action that pulls and propels people in multiple directions' (Musolino, Warin and Gilchrist 2018: 546). In my fieldwork in nursing homes, staff would often expand on the fixed and singular way of understanding not eating by considering the ambiguities and multiple meanings of this distressing phenomenon and experiment with the possibilities of delivering care to relieve their sufferings. Some methods of feeding, as the next section will show, work better than others.

## Caring at the Threshold of Life and Death

Most of the personal care workers who attempted to feed Mrs Brie failed. She regularly closed her mouth to food and rapidly lost weight. Staff drew the conclusion that, due to the progression of her dementia, she was no longer aware of her need to eat and had no interest in food. Maureen, a veteran personal care worker disagreed with them. For Maureen, it was important not to assume that Mrs Brie did not want to eat. She may, as Maureen suggested, just be *not prepared* for eating. 'You can't go straight to the task [of feeding],' Maureen said. 'She needs to prepare herself for it [eating].' When I asked her, Maureen explained what she meant here by the word 'prepare'.

For residents who feed themselves, eating is not a straightforward process. Their sense of eating is made in and through the movements involved in each phase, from preparing to eat to transferring, chewing and swallowing. The idea of consuming food, the smell of food and even the trip leading to the dining area all prepare them for eating. Well before food is transferred from plate to mouth, bodies adjust to support an 'openness' to the food on offer. It starts from the multisensory processes of incorporation – inspecting the dish (appealing or repellent), smelling the aroma (familiar or strange), feeling the plate (hot, warm or cold) and handling the cutlery – before getting even the first mouthful of food. The movements of hands and fingers, the touch and temperature of utensils, and the sight and smell of food all lead to a sense of craving, then an understanding of the situation, and then a response: opening the mouth as food is transferred from plate to mouth. Residents in late-stage dementia may have lost the capacity to respond to what may seem like a strange situation having food delivered to their mouths on a spoon. In the case of Mrs Brie, she needed to be 'attuned'. She could not open her mouth at will. Someone needed to get her started. To prepare for eating, Mrs Brie needed staff assistance.

To illustrate, Maureen once showed me how she usually assisted Mrs Brie with her lunch in the open dining area of the facility. Maureen first checked that Mrs Brie was wearing her glasses and hearing aids. 'She may not be able to understand what I say to her,' Maureen said, 'but at least then she can hear my voice and see what is coming on the spoon. Not being able to see and hear can be scary for residents, which adds to their confusion.' Seating herself lower so as to face Mrs Brie at eye level, Maureen drew her attention by gently holding her hands in her own. 'It's time for lunch, Mrs Brie.' Maureen spoke calmly and gave Mrs Brie a little hand massage. Once Mrs Brie lifted her head and fixed her eyes on her, Maureen adjusted the princess chair so that she was sitting upright with her head inclined forwards. Maureen continued: 'If the resident is drowsy, she may struggle to swallow safely. Before offering food and drink, I make sure they are alert, comfortable and sitting upright.' Remember that Mrs Brie's drowsiness was caused by the antipsychotic medication as well as her diminished ability to connect consciously with others. In preparing Mrs Brie through touch and the adjustment of her posture, Maureen's care counteracted the medication-induced drowsiness and increased Mrs Brie's possibility of connectedness with other material things in her environment.

What Maureen did to get Mrs Brie 'started' demonstrates that simple attentional and postural adjustments could help her to incorporate food into her body. Posture is important while eating. Sitting up and tilting the head forwards while swallowing will help protect the airway. Mrs Brie seemed to become attentive towards Maureen, shown through how she slightly tilted and turned her head to follow Maureen's movements. As Mrs Brie became increasingly aware of the presence and movements of Maureen, a friendly and comforting other person, Mrs Brie could prepare herself for a further connection with food and the multisensory experience of eating.

How Maureen assisted Mrs Brie with her preparation for eating reveals a process, as Maureen said, of 'wakening up' a body so that connections and extensions can be created. Though moving food into and through the body is ordinarily experienced as sensory by nature, without conscious attention, for residents like Mrs Brie, sensuous stimuli from other persons was a way to trigger more intense sensorial arousal, which could prepare her for eating and drinking. However, in the case of most residents who were fed by staff, that process of preparing them for opening the mouth and eating was often absent. Sadly, residents were sometimes expected to start eating just as soon as staff started feeding them, with no thought given to their readiness or otherwise. According to my observations, meals were often left to sit in front of residents when staff had difficulty in feeding them and trays were then removed with the food almost untouched.

Still sitting in Mrs Brie's line of sight, Maureen started helping Mrs Brie with her lunch as she explained further: 'Residents with dementia like Mrs Brie do not open the mouth if staff feed them straightaway. They need to be reminded to open the mouth to take in food and then close the mouth to swallow.' Mrs Brie may not have been able to understand the situation cognitively, as people ordinarily do, due to her advanced dementia, but clearly she could become *sensuously* attuned to it. Using a small teaspoon, Maureen touched Mrs Brie's lower lip with the tip of the spoon and waited for Mrs Brie to open her mouth. Mrs Brie then opened a tiny gap between her lips. Maureen then carefully introduced two small teaspoons of ice cream through the gap. For some residents, reduced or thicker saliva might make the mouth dry, increasing swallowing difficulty. Ice cream can both ease the sensation of dryness in the mouth and activate the taste buds. Mrs Brie tilted her head a little further back while holding the ice cream in her mouth. I could see a clear swallowing motion of her throat after a few seconds.

As I described earlier in this chapter, Mrs Brie could, in earlier days, eat and enjoy home-baked apple pie using her fingers. This shows how a productive desire can be ignited by encountering the sensory properties of familiar food. Bodily parts and material things – for example, the hands, mouth, lipped plate and feeder cup – are pulled in to trigger a productive desire. Maureen showed me how she prepared Mrs Brie for eating: a motion of the mouth and movements of the tongue were triggered by a gentle touch on the lip and a teaspoonful of ice cream. The coolness and sweetness of the ice cream teased the taste buds as it dissolved, resulting in a tongue that could twist, a mouth that could open and a body that could eat. Mrs Brie was ready to have her meal.

Filling the teaspoon, this time with a tiny amount of pureed beef, Maureen lifted the spoon in front of Mrs Brie's left eye and then almost immediately lowered the spoon to her mouth. Mrs Brie did not open her mouth. Maureen then repeated her previous movements: positioned the spoon in front of her left eye for two seconds and then lowered the spoon to the mouth. This time Mrs Brie opened her mouth. Maureen inserted the teaspoon flat into the gap between her lips and then lifted the handle of the spoon to form a sharp angle so that the pureed beef could slide neatly into her mouth. Intrigued by this routine, I asked Maureen why she put the spoon first in front of Mrs Brie's left eye and not directly into her mouth. Maureen explained: 'Mrs Brie has zero vision on her right eye and the vision on her left eye is limited. I need to show her the food on the spoon so that she understands that I am feeding her and opens her mouth to eat.'

To prompt Mrs Brie to make a swallowing motion, Maureen used the fingertips of her left hand, gently tapping on Mrs Brie's throat. 'Swallow', Maureen said. She then pressed her lips together and made a swallowing motion in her own throat. 'Swallow', she repeated. She looked closely at Mrs Brie's face and throat, for signs of swallowing. The fine muscles around Mrs Brie's mouth tightened, while she half-closed her eyes and slightly tilted her head. There was a visible undulation of her throat as the meat travelled down through her epiglottis. Spoon by spoon, Maureen and Mrs Brie repeated, in turn, their respective roles in the sequence of movements of assisted eating. I asked how she knew whether Mrs Brie was full or not. 'She pushes out the spoon, using her tongue, and seals her lips,' and Maureen demonstrated, pressing her lips tightly together.

In Deleuze and Guattari's theories of desiring-production, a 'line of flight' (1988) works to break open existing structures and create new connections in a productive process of change and morphosis. For residents living the tension between eating and not eating, there exists a threshold of intensities that can lead up to a change from not eating to eating. A trigger, the sight of other people eating or the sensation of the sweetness and coolness of ice cream may work like a line of flight, inducing changes in sensory intensities, leading to a threshold between the opposing bodily states of eating or not eating. When a relational process (seeing people eating or swallowing ice cream) is triggered, it instantly creates a type of connection between person and food capable of changing a person's mode of being and ways of relating in the world. This demonstrates that from eating to not eating there is a certain turning point or threshold over which we can make a crossing. Once residents have been attuned by staff to become ready to open their mouths, the unproductive state of not eating can be converted into a productive process of eating.

However, it is also important to note that the discomfort induced by swallowing difficulty can be another dimension involved in residents' eating. Also, a certain trigger, such as a lump of undercooked potato or a soup that is spicy, may induce choking or coughing, physical reactions that are counterproductive to the experience of eating. A productive process of eating can sometimes be reversed in such situations when discomfiture becomes intense and residents may stop eating to avoid it. Triggering is concerned with the movements of a productive desire as multiplicities; it is an intensity that goes in many different directions and produces openings and closures, as well as possibilities of 'becomings'. This leads to the understanding that the right care for residents with eating difficulties cannot be prescriptive; it involves experimenting and always being prepared to adapt to ambiguities and ambivalences.

A right assemblage of care can help to overcome the challenges posed by residents' eating difficulties, be it in the form of a choking risk or residents closing their mouths to food. Nevertheless, as this chapter has shown using the example of Mrs Brie, what was considered as 'care' that was prescribed to protect Mrs Brie from choking – namely, a vitaminized diet – had led her to stop eating altogether, become malnourished and lose weight. As a practice of nutritional care, is this provision of texture-modified food the right care for Mrs Brie if it leads to her malnutrition? The change of her diet from soft to vitaminized marked a tipping point, not only in her choice of food but also in her lunch routine with Heather and her experience of eating. In receiving her altered nutrition, Mrs Brie could hardly feel any sense of connectedness, comfort or being cared for.

In terms of policy, by adhering to dysphagia management procedures, the service providers are complying with the Australian Aged Care Quality Standards. No provider wants to be found liable for a death that is deemed 'preventable'. They need to show that they followed guidelines and took precautions, even if it means providing food that residents may reject. On the other hand, the Dietitians Association of Australia (2019: 12) asserts that the prevalence of malnutrition among nursing home residents reflects a systemic failure that is not being addressed by current practice and accreditation standards. As the current accreditation process focuses on monitoring compliance rather than quality improvement (Productivity Commission 2011b: 101), service providers choose to foreground risk of residents choking rather than the underlying risk of death by malnutrition, in order to reduce their own risk of liability.

Ironically, as observed in the nursing homes, inadequate assistance from staff for residents who need supervised support with eating and drinking is very relevant to *both* residents' risk of choking and their longer-term risk of malnutrition and dehydration. Regardless of diet, a resident deemed at risk of choking needs to be supervised while eating to ensure their safety and adequate intake. For residents who have eating difficulties, physical assistance with eating and drinking needs to be performed by personal care workers, which also reduces residents' choking risk. Aged care service providers are actually subsidized more money per day if the resident is assessed as requiring staff supervision or assistance with eating and drinking. However, as Dietitians Association of Australia reports, some providers who have been allocated the funding do not provide the higher level of assistance to their residents. My fieldwork in the nursing homes indicates that this is often due to the low staffing level. In one facility, care staff constantly told me that they are too busy to take the extra time it requires to feed residents who are 'picky', too slow, or who close their mouths to food, as they have 'too many other residents to feed'. While attending to residents at mealtimes, some carers appeared not to notice the poor intake of nourishment. Fluids were often left to the residents, even when they were unable to hold a cup or needed prompts to drink. If residents with late-stage dementia and swallowing difficulties are to be assisted to eat, through a right assemblage of care, the focus in policy and practice needs to shift to centre the needs and preferences of residents and the concerns of their family and friends.

Dying residents may experience neither a need to eat nor an appetite for food. For these residents, there is no sense in taking in food: the body is losing connections, and its final dispersal is imminent. Dying brings about the end of the breathing, sensing and feeling body. Mrs Brie died during my fieldwork. As death approached, her breathing became laboured. With increasing weakness and fatigue, she eventually stopped eating and drinking altogether, and slept most of the time. Heather consented for her mother to receive palliative care. Mrs Brie's care plan was then adjusted. As part of her palliative care plan, a routine was set up to reposition her in bed regularly to prevent pressure sores and to give oral hygiene, consisting of oral swabs and lubricants to relieve her dry mouth. A syringe driver, a small portable device that administers medicines subcutaneously over a selected time period, was also used for her pain management. It was the easiest way to administer the pain medication that Mrs Brie needed to stay comfortable during her process of dying.

Saddened that the life of her mother was approaching its end, Heather came to see Mrs Brie every day and spent long periods sitting at her bedside. 'Dying must be hard,' Heather said, hearing her mother's laboured breathing and seeing her chest visibly rising and falling under the white bedsheet. Studies on elderly people's experience of dying in nursing homes highlight the discomfort of dying, reporting that residents often experience pain, pressure sores and thirst, as well as loneliness and depression (Greenwood et al. 2018; McNamara 2001).

Between stopping to eat and taking the last breath, life lingers at its own pace. For nursing home residents with late-stage dementia, living with profound impairments and dying with pain are both difficult life situations. The right care for these residents is thus to care for their chance to live a good life during their last years or months and then to die a good death. In both living and dying, caring for these residents is a matter of attending to them, responding to their innermost drives and trying to meet their needs. Right care at the end of life is thus associated with relief from suffering and a sense of peace as a person faces imminent death.

Once death arrives, movement stops. No longer propelled to walk or eat, one's sensation of pleasure and exercise of autonomy are irrevocably lost. Yet, with right assemblages of care residents may be assisted, accompanied and comforted to feel at ease and at home right up until the final moment.

## Note

1. Savishinsky (2003) describes how feeding is carried out by staff almost as if they were just filling a container, with residents passive and submissive. For Savishinsky, food is a powerful entrance into aged care practices; he explores the meanings of food in the institution and the ways in which it is entwined with issues of conflict and control. Yet, as this chapter illustrates, even for the most severely impaired residents, eating cannot be reduced to a mechanical process of stuffing. A body that eats is attentive, responsive and productive. Eating is always an event and a process in which a body connects and extends.

# CONCLUSION

## Becoming Ethical through Care

As stated in the Introduction to this book, the rationale of today's dementia diagnosis highlights loss – brain damage and cognitive decline, and the associated disabilities of being unable to remember, reflect on or recognize objects and persons, or communicate using language. This medicalized rationale leads to disease-centred dementia care, where lived experiences of people with dementia are understood and treated as symptoms. In Chapters 1 to 4, we considered how the walking of residents during the later stages of dementia was medically constructed into 'wandering' and their movements as 'agitation', and thereby classified under the behavioural and psychological symptoms of dementia. We took as examples the walking of Mrs Sage, who had Alzheimer's disease, the attempted standing and walking of Mr Dixon, who had dementia with Lewy bodies, and Mr Harris, who had dementia associated with his Parkinson's disease. These examples demonstrated, in terms of care practices, that when bodies are labelled as mindless or moving meaninglessly, this leads to restrictive practices of risk minimization. Such practices include the use of bodily restraints that prevent standing or walking, leading to detrimental effects on residents' quality of life.

The clear message of this book is that residents' movements of walking, of standing and of eating are important: they are intrinsic to their possibilities to extend, connect and feel at home in the nursing home. This presents a challenge to the many biomedical assumptions and clinical constructions of movement that are based on a cognitive-centred understanding of personhood. Strongly criticizing the cognitive-centred conception of personhood, Tom Kitwood argued that the person living with dementia is still a human being, who 'is still an agent, one who can make things happen in the world, a sentient, relational and historical being' (Kitwood 1993: 541). He redefines personhood as 'a standing or status that is bestowed upon one human being by others in the context of relationship and social being', stressing the qualities of 'recognition, respect and trust' (Kitwood 1997: 8). The notion that a patient with dementia will *still* be a person if they are *related to* by other people and *recognized as* a person is central to Kitwood's theorization of person-centred care.

In nursing homes, the discourse of person-centred dementia care, opposing the disease-centred dementia care approach, is increasingly emphasized in staff training to bring changes to staff attitudes and care practices. A key ethical principle in Dementia Dynamics (person-centred care) training is to recognize that a patient with dementia is still a person who is 'no different to you and me' in terms of human value and human rights. It was written into the handouts of training sessions that I attended in my fieldwork, and I quote:

> Every person has the right to enjoy the freedom to fully participate in life, regardless of their disabilities. No disability can take away your dignity or value as a human being. The person lying in a fallout chair who cannot speak, or eat without help, who can't take themselves to the toilet or let you know what they need, or can't walk about anymore – that person has the same human value as you and me.

The assertion that people with dementia are 'no different to you and me' sends a powerful message in terms of advocating for residents' rights and how these may influence care practices. Staff at sessions I attended talked insightfully in chats during the intervals about how aged residents they cared for often related to people around them in different ways. One female care worker said:

> Sometimes families are angry at us. They say we don't care, and treat residents like objects. I thought the same before I worked this job. Now I know it's not always about treating residents like objects. My Nanny is the same age as [many of] the old people living here, and I treat residents like they are my own old people. [But] sometimes it's hard to relate to residents who are completely mute and have 'behaviours'. I want to help but don't understand what they want.

How residents with advanced dementia relate to other people and how those ways of relating may tend to change due to their conditions does have an impact on the delivery of their daily care. For example, I once heard Mrs Anderson calling out 'Help!', 'Help!' from her room. I found a carer and told her that Mrs Anderson might need urgent help. The carer looked unconcerned and said to me: 'She does that all the time just to get people's attention. You can sit with her if you like, or I will check on her before handover.' She then added, 'Mrs Casey can't find her new blouse and asked me to call the laundry. I'd better go to find her blouse before she complains to the RN.' Although shocked by the carer's indifference, I was not surprised by her dismissive attitude to Mrs Anderson's calling for help. On several occasions similar to this one, I was told by staff that residents with late-stage dementia like Mrs Anderson 'do not *really* want anything'. My observations are in line with findings from Jackson's study on routinized and extra care. Staff would more often direct their assistance to those residents 'to whom a staff member felt connected'. The extra, informal care is provided 'less frequently to patients that a staff member related to only with difficulty' (E. Jackson 1997: 198).

To overcome this difficulty in relating to residents with advanced dementia, staff made efforts to utilize the person-centred dementia care approach in daily care practices. An example may be seen in how staff sought meaning in Mrs Sage's wandering. The nursing team believed that Mrs Sage's excessive walking must be purposeful, although obviously affected by her dementia. Finally, they agreed that Mrs Sage must have been in search of something or someone in her past. They worked diligently through the medical records, life histories and chats with Mrs Sage's loved ones in the hope of rediscovering the *real* Mrs Sage, the person hidden within the construct of 'person with dementia', and specifically, what kind of search it was that drove her tireless walking. The nursing team here demonstrated the underlying assumption that people with dementia must always have an aim and purpose in what they do, just like them, and in doing so were trying to impose meaning on Mrs Sage's walking.

As described in Chapter 2, residents like Mrs Sage made sense of material things and persons in and through immediate and spontaneous encounters. For these residents, it was not the meaning but the multisensory extensions and correspondence with other material things and persons that gave them a sense of rightness of 'being-in-the-world-with-others'. Although suffering an 'absent mind' due to cognitive changes, their *movements* were still sensible and productive in the Deleuzian sense to enable them, by extension, to feel at home in the nursing home. Equally important to the recognition of residents with dementia as being no different to other people in terms of human value and human rights, we must also understand and address their *differences* in their ways of relating to other things and beings in their world.

Janelle Taylor, an anthropologist whose mother had Alzheimer's and lived in a nursing home, recognized her mother as still 'in many ways the cheerful, affectionate person' that she enjoyed being with. Janelle thought about this in terms of many 'stills' and 'firsts'; for example, 'The first time she tried to sign her own name and could not. The first time she needed my help in the shower' (2008: 316). Despite all the changes her mother had been through, she maintained their close relationship through walks that they shared and chats that they exchanged. Although recalling all those painful 'firsts', Janelle sought to relate with her mother by finding the 'stills', which reminded her that being-in-the-world with others continues in the face of the debilitating effects of disease. The progress of her mother's dementia made it difficult for her to comprehend the suffering of those around her, 'but she still does notice and respond to others and is still moved to try to alleviate their distress' (2008: 329). At the core of how Janelle related to her mother, then, was walking alongside her and finding the *stills* – those things that people with dementia are still capable of doing and enjoying – and always joining her mother in activities that they could still share, such as having a conversation or walking.

Drawing on the ethnographic case studies presented in this book, I conclude that despite cognitive changes, as well bodily impairments, productive conditions, lived by residents as the stills, could be found to help residents move, extend their possibilities and ultimately enable them to feel at home in the nursing home. This study contributes new knowledge about how people with dementia can still relate to other things and persons, not cognitively, perhaps, but sensorially and affectively. To create the right care for people who suffer from dementia, biomedical constructs of resident movement need to be challenged to foreground the 'stills': what can still be productive possibilities in creating multisensory connections and affective relations between people with dementia and those who move alongside and care for them.

# EPILOGUE

In walking, caring or doing research, we are all connected in one way or another in a quest to create a sense of home. On those long days of fieldwork, as I walked up and down the corridors of the nursing homes, immersed in and touched by their sights, smells and sounds, my heart would often sink and my legs would grow heavy. Images of home and my father and mother came flashing back. My father was diagnosed with Alzheimer's in 2000. He was cared for at home by my mum, with love and dedication. He died at dawn, on 26 January 2010 in Beijing, China. My brother sat up on his last night, holding his hands until the very last moment of his life. I was not there for his departure, but in walking alongside nursing home residents and later writing this book, I felt him with me. I came to realize that writing this ethnography is how I have created a sense of home away from home, even as I tried to hold on to my Mum and Dad and the time that we shared. My effort to hold on is doomed to fail as, like everyone else, I am ageing and will eventually decline and die. However, during my finite life I cannot help but strive to constantly remake a sense of home. That sense of home can come, as this book shows, when we hold on to each other to give and receive right care. Only in so doing does life become bearable and meaningful.

# AFTERWORD

## Philip B. Stafford

Some twenty-five years ago, my friend and colleague, Jody Curley, led elderly day care participants in a discussion of the concept of home, as part of a wider community study of the experience of place. She synthesized their evocative expressions into a collective poem called Home, as follows:

***Home***
*I have several homes*
*I know a home is a home when I can*
*Go there*
*And go out again.*
*Home is where the dog goes*
*When it gets too cold to roam*
*When winter's coming on*
*That's when I want to go*
*Home.*

The poem is rarely far from both my personal and my professional perspectives on the world, on the changes in my own life and from my personal philosophy of living. That's why I was delighted to be contacted by Dr Zhang, who felt the poem deserved some attention within the frame of her wonderful book, which you, dear reader, have just finished.

I am amazed at the startling correspondence of assertions between Dr Zhang's ethnographic research and the assertions offered by a group of elderly, mostly demented women in Bloomington, Indiana. I feel it provides a compelling and perhaps universal affirmation of the findings in the study. In simple terms, it echoes three conclusions reached by Dr Zhang.

*I have several homes*: home is not tied to a singular, bricks and mortar structure or place-specific objects.

> Conceptualizing home in terms of household objects, which must, by definition, relate to domestic objects in residents' rooms, can be simplistic and reductive, as that definition cannot accommodate the complex and productive interrelationships between residents and other people and fittings in the

> wider nursing home environment, such as carpeted floors, grab-rails and corridors. … the feeling of being-at-home emerges through the lived experience of being in contact with other people and other objects in the nursing home.

*… a home is a home when I can go there and go out again*: home is the fulcrum of our daily experience and enters into our lives not because of its stasis but, rather, its dynamism. To occupy a home is to be 'doing home', as Zhang refers to it, or homemaking in my own writing about the concept. In the nursing home, movement is institutionally valued, albeit clinically constructed as 'ambulation' in treatment plans. Zhang unpacks the notion of movement to first principles, agreeing with Ingold that movement is life – *movimiento es vida* – and then she writes: 'I hold the view that life continues across home and the nursing home not because of particular possessions, persons or practices but because, even in care, people continue to live their everyday lives through walking, standing and eating – the ordinary daily movements that are fundamental to our being-in-the-world.'

Zhang offers great insight into the phenomenon of wandering in the nursing home by distinguishing wandering from walking, where walking, after Ingold and others …

> In a coordinated natural flow, all Mrs Sage's bodily movements, including those involved in walking, are operating in the dimension of instrumental attention or 'subsidiary awareness', to use Polanyi's term. This leads her to be able to 'feel' what is around her through the positions and movements of her body parts. Merging the matrix of sensory properties of place with her 'feeling awareness' of the exterior world, Mrs Sage was kept alive in a web of connectedness. In and through walking, Mrs Sage weaved herself into the lived fabric of the nursing home environment … For nursing home residents with dementia, the act of walking should never be reduced to a symptom of brain pathology. Instead, in and through walking, they could discover and re-create a sense of home.

*Home is where the dog goes when it gets too cold to roam. When winter's coming on, that's when I want to go home*: The participants assert that they share the homing instincts of dogs and, I believe, capture the metaphor of old age as the winter of our lives. This is not meant to trivialize the metaphor, which must strain against its ubiquitous use in literature and, sadly, its monetization in marketing ventures designed to pitch a retirement of sunny climes and sunburnt skin. For me, the image of a dog settling on the fireplace rug by circling in smaller and smaller circles until a centre is found evokes exactly the to and fro, back and forth movement of going out and coming back – the bare, *urform* of movement that Zhang refers to throughout her work. To me, it seems fair to refer to movement as a life force that springs from a need and, as Jean Piaget argued, represents the first developmental stage of life and, as I infer from Zhang, perhaps the last.

*At Home in a Nursing Home*, of course, covers a great deal more territory than the three simple thoughts expressed in the poem – home is not the house; home is a verb, home is going out and coming back. This small group of elderly people with dementia demonstrates the profound wisdom to be found in people stripped of convention, of rationalization, of self-objectification. For elders with dementia, metaphor becomes the lovely medium taken up for expression, not purposely for artistic effect but as an alternative way of using language to be in the world. Unlike the representational function of simile, metaphor creates meaning through fusing previously unrelatable elements; Zhang, following Deleuze, argues that 'right care' consists of the creation of assemblages that fuse the elements of human capability (in the face of deterioration) and complementary support (whether human or technological).

**Philip B. Stafford** is a cultural anthropologist, with a BA from the University of Chicago and Ph.D. from Indiana University. For forty years, Phil has focused his efforts on the creation of age- and ability-friendly communities. He has consulted and published widely on the relationship between aging and place, with publications including *Gray Areas: Ethnographic Encounters with Nursing Home Culture* (2003), *Elderburbia: Aging with a Sense of Place in America* (2009) *and The Global Age-Friendly Community Movement: A Critical Perspective* (2018).

# GLOSSARY

**Assemblage**: A key concept for Deleuze and Guattari (1988) to seek to account for change in becomings in which objects, beings, events, processes and discourses of heterogenous natures co-exist as multiplicities through metamorphosis.

**Being-at-home-in-the-world**: To speak of 'at-homeness', Michael Jackson suggests that people everywhere try to strike a balance between closure and openness, between acting and being acted upon, between acquiescing to the given and choosing their own fate.

**Becoming-at-home-in-the-world**: This notion is used in this book to shift the focus from conscious experience of a sense of home to its constitution in the preconscious productive processes.

**Correspondence**: Tim Ingold's notion of correspondence describes dynamic processes of engaging with other material things and beings in and through movements.

**Doing undergoing**: In Dewey's terms, the doing is also an undergoing; what we do is also done in us. To experience is to engage in a process of doing and undergoing.

**Habit**: Drawing on the work of John Dewey, Tim Ingold argues for an understanding of habit that rests on the way in which the practitioner, while actively engaged in the practice, is inside it. In dwelling in-habit, improvisation and experience come together in a forwarding and open-ended process as one.

**Lifeworld**: A fundamental concept in phenomenology; the world of lived experience inhabited by humans as conscious beings.

**Line of flight**: A line of flight is a concept developed by Gilles Deleuze and Félix Guattari in their work *Capitalism and Schizophrenia*. It describes how a factor in an assemblage ultimately allows it to change and adapt to said changes.

**Multiplicity**: A Deleuze concept that describes a complex that does not refer to a prior unity. A situation is an ensemble of different assemblages of things, persons, processes, discourses and practices that emerge and actualize into movements, against a background of ever-changing circumstances.

# REFERENCES


Adam, Barbara. 1995. *Timewatch: The Social Analysis of Time*. New Jersey: Wiley.

Adolph, Karen E., et al. 2012. 'How Do You Learn to Walk? Thousands of Steps and Dozens of Falls Per Day', *Psychological Science* 23: 1387–94.

Ahmed, Sara. 1999. 'Home and Away: Narratives of Migration and Estrangement', *International Journal of Cultural Studies* 2: 329–47.

Algase, Donna L., et al. 1996. 'Need-Driven Dementia-Compromised Behavior: An Alternative View of Disruptive Behavior', *American Journal of Alzheimer's Disease* 11: 10–19.

Algase, Donna L., et al. 2007. 'Mapping the Maze of Terms and Definitions in Dementia-Related Wandering', *Aging & Mental Health* 11: 686–98.

Allan, Graham, and Graham Crow (eds). 1989. *Home and Family: Creating the Domestic Sphere*. Basingstoke, UK: Palgrave Macmillan.

Australian Bureau of Statistics (ABS). 1988. 'History of Pensions and Other Benefits in Australia'. Canberra: Australian Bureau of Statistics. Retrieved 14 August 2020 from https://www.abs.gov.au/ausstats/abs@.nsf/94713ad445ff1425ca25682000192af2/8e72c4526a94aaedca2569de00296978!opendocument.

———. 2016. 'Disability, Ageing and Carers, Australia: Summary of Findings, 2015'. Canberra: Australian Bureau of Statistics. Retrieved 28 November 2021 from https://www.abs.gov.au/AUSSTATS/abs@.nsf/Previousproducts/4430.0Main%20Features302015?opendocument&tabname=Summary&prodno=4430.0&issue=2015&num=&view.

Australian Institute of Health and Welfare (AIHW). 2002. 'Ageing in Place: Before and After the 1997 Aged Care Reforms'. Australian Institute of Health & Welfare.

———. 2007. 'Dementia in Australia: National Data Analysis and Development'. Canberra: Australian Institute of Health and Welfare.

———. 2012. 'Residential Aged Care in Australia 2010–11: A Statistical Overview'. *Aged Care Statistics Series No. 36. Cat. No. AGE 68*. Canberra: Australian Institute of Health and Welfare.

Australian Nursing and Midwifery Federation (ANMF). 2019. ANMF National Aged Care Survey 2019 – Final Report. Melbourne, Victoria.

Ballenger, Jesse F. 2006. 'The Biomedical Deconstruction of Senility and the Persistent Stigmatization of Old Age in the United States', in Annette Leibing and Lawrence Cohen (eds), *Thinking about Dementia: Culture, Loss, and the Anthropology of Senility*. New Brunswick, NJ: Rutgers University Press, pp. 106–20.

Barbaras, Renaud. 2008. 'Life, Movement, and Desire', *Research in Phenomenology* 38: 3–17.
Bauman, Zygmunt. 1991. *Modernity and Ambivalence*. Cambridge: Polity Press.
Bergman, Howard, et al. 2007. 'Frailty: An Emerging Research and Clinical Paradigm – Issues and Controversies', *The Journals of Gerontology: Series A* 62: 731–37.
Bland, Marian. 2003. 'All the Comforts of Home? A Critical Ethnography of Residential Aged Care in New Zealand', Ph.D. dissertation, University of Newcastle.
———. 2007. 'Betwixt and Between: A Critical Ethnography of Comfort in New Zealand Residential Aged Care', *Journal of Clinical Nursing* 16: 937–44.
Brett, Lindsey, Victoria Traynor and Paul Stapley. 2016. 'Effects of Physical Exercise on Health and Well-Being of Individuals Living with a Dementia in Nursing Homes: A Systematic Review', *Journal of the American Medical Directors Association* 17: 104–16.
Brodaty, Henry, Brian Draper and Lee-Fay Low. 2003. 'Behavioural and Psychological Symptoms of Dementia: A Seven-Tiered Model of Service Delivery', *Medical Journal of Australia* 178: 231–34.
Cheu, Sandy. 2018. 'New Analysis Indicates Staffing Ratios in Aged Care also Provide Economic Benefits', *Australian Ageing Agenda*. Retrieved 18 August 2020 from https://www.australianageingagenda.com.au/executive/new-analysis-indicates-staffing-ratios-in-aged-care-also-provide-economic-benefits/.
Cohen, Lawrence. 1998. *No Aging in India: Alzheimer's, the Bad Family, and other Modern Things*. Berkeley: University of California Press.
———. 2006. 'Introduction', in Annette Leibing and Lawrence Cohen (eds), *Thinking about Dementia: Culture, Loss, the Anthropology of Senility*. New Brunswick, NJ: Rutgers University Press, pp. 1–19.
Cram, Fiona, and Helen Paton. 1993. 'Personal Possessions and Self-identity: The Experiences of Elderly Women in Three Residential Settings', *Australian Journal on Ageing* 12: 19–24.
DeForge, Ryan et al. 2011. 'Afraid to Care; Unable to Care: A Critical Ethnography within a Long-Term Care Home', *Journal of Ageing Studies* 25: 415–26.
Deleuze, Gilles, and Félix Guattari. 1977. *Anti-Oedipus: Capitalism and Schizophrenia*. New York: The Viking Press.
———. 1988. *A Thousand Plateaus: Capitalism and Schizophrenia*. London: The Athlone Press.
Dennis, Simone. 2004. 'Melted Honey: Sax and Sex', *Popular Culture Review* 15: 47–61.
———. 2007. *Police Beat: The Emotional Power of Music in Police Work*. NY: Cambria Press.
———. 2018. 'Analysing Smokefree: Notes on Senses, Smoke and Violence', *Anthropological Forum* 28: 171–82.
Den Ouden, Mirre, et al. 2015. 'Daily (In)Activities of Nursing Home Residents in Their Wards: An Observation Study', *Journal of the American Medical Directors Association* 16: 963–68.
Department of Health. 2019. '6th Report on Funding and Financing of the Aged Care Sector', July 2018. Canberra.
———. 2020. 'Extra Services Agreements for Residential Aged Care'. Retrieved 19 July 2020 from https://www.health.gov.au/initiatives-and-programs/residential-aged-

care/managing-residential-aged-care-services/extra-services-agreements-for-residential-aged-care.

Department of Health and Ageing. 2012a. 'Decision-Making Tool: Supporting a Restraint Free Environment in Residential Aged Care'. Canberra: Department of Health and Ageing.

———. 2012b. 'Living Longer, Living Better: Aged Care Reform Package'. Canberra: Department of Health and Aging.

———. 2013. 'Aged Care Funding Instrument User Guide'. Canberra: Department of Health and Aging.

Dewey, John. 2015. *Experience and Education*. New York: Free Press.

Diamond, Timothy. 1992. *Making Gray Gold: Narratives of Nursing Home Care*. Chicago, IL: University of Chicago Press.

Dietitians Association of Australia. 2019. 'Submission to Royal Commission into Aged Care Quality and Safety'. Retrieved 4 January 2022 from https://dietitiansaustralia.org.au/wp-content/uploads/2019/03/DAA_Royal-Commission-Aged-Care_Mar-2019_Final.pdf.

Fiveash, Barb. 1998. 'The Experience of Nursing Home Life', *International Journal of Nursing Practice* 4: 166–74.

Förstl, Hans, and Alexander Kurz. 1999. 'Clinical Features of Alzheimer's Disease', *European Archives of Psychiatry and Clinical Neuroscience* 249: 288–90.

Foucault, Michel. 1980. *The History of Sexuality. Volume 1: An Introduction*. Harmondsworth, UK: Penguin.

———. 2012. *Discipline and Punish: The Birth of the Prison*. New York: Vintage.

Fox, Nicholas. 2012. *The Body*. Cambridge: Polity Press.

Gault, Mandy L., and Mark E.T Willems. 2013. 'Aging, Functional Capacity and Eccentric Exercise Training', *Aging and Disease* 4: 351.

George, Karen, and Gary George. 2011. 'Destitute Asylum (1851 – c. 1917)'. Retrieved 19 July 2020 from https://www.findandconnect.gov.au/ref/sa/biogs/SE00062b.htm.

Giannouli, Eleftheria, et al. 2016. 'Mobility in Old Age: Capacity is Not Performance', *BioMed Research International 2016*.

Goffman, Erving. 1961. *Asylums: Essays on the Social Situation of Mental Patients and Other Innates*. New York: Anchor Books/Doubleday.

Greenwood, Nan, et al. 2018. 'Experiences of Older People Dying in Nursing Homes: A Narrative Systematic Review of Qualitative Studies', *BMJ Open* 8.

Groves, Aaron, et al. 2017. The Oakden Report. Adelaide, South Australia: SA Health, Department for Health and Ageing.

Gubrium, Jaber F. 1975. *Living and Dying at Murray Manor*. New York: St. Martin's Press.

———. 1993. *Speaking of Life: Horizons of Meaning for Nursing Home Residents*. New Jersey: Transaction Publishers.

Guen, Roxane L. 1993. 'Residential Care for the Aged: An Overview of Government Policy from 1962 to 1993'. Canberra: Parliament of the Commonwealth of Australia.

Gurney, Craig M. 1997. '"... Half of Me Was Satisfied": Making Sense of Home through Episodic Ethnographies', *Women's Studies International Forum* 20(3): 373–86.

Harbers, Hans, Annemarie Mol and Alice Stollmeyer. 2002. 'Food Matters', *Theory, Culture & Society* 19: 207–26.

Harnett, Tove. 2010. 'Seeking Exemptions from Nursing Home Routines: Residents' Everyday Influence Attempts and Institutional Order', *Journal of Aging Studies* 24: 292–301.

Henderson, Neil. 2003. 'Alzheimer's Units and Special Care: A Soteriological Fantasy', in Philip Stafford (ed.), *Gray Areas: Ethnographic Encounters with Nursing Home Culture*. Santa Fe, NM: School of American Research Press, pp. 153–72.

Higgins, J. 1989. 'Homes and Institutions', in Graham Allan and Graham Crow (eds), *Home and Family: Creating the Domestic Sphere*. UK: Palgrave Macmillan.

High, Dallas M., and Graham D. Rowles. 1995. 'Nursing Home Residents, Families, and Decision Making: Toward an Understanding of Progressive Surrogacy', *Journal of Aging Studies* 9: 101–17.

Hugo, Cherie, et al. 2018. 'What Does it Cost to Feed Aged Care Residents in Australia?', *Nutrition & Dietetics* 75: 6–10.

Hull, William, et al. 1863. 'Report of the Commissioners Appointed to Enquire into the Municipalities and Charitable Institutions of Victoria'. Melbourne: Parliament of Victoria.

Ibrahim, Joseph E., et al. 2017. 'Premature Deaths of Nursing Home Residents: An Epidemiological Analysis', *Medical Journal of Australia* 206: 442–47.

Ijaopo, Ezekiel. O. 2017. 'Dementia-Related Agitation: A Review of Non-pharmacological Interventions and Analysis of Risks and Benefits of Pharmacotherapy', *Translational Psychiatry* 7(10): e1250.

Ingold, Tim. 2011. *Being Alive: Essays on Movement, Knowledge and Description*. Oxfordshire: Routledge.

———. 2017. 'On Human Correspondence', *Journal of the Royal Anthropological Institute* 23: 9–27.

———. 2022. *Being Alive: Essays on Movement, Knowledge and Description*. London & New York: Routledge.

Ingold, Tim, and Elizabeth Hallam. 2007. 'Creativity and Cultural Improvisation: An Introduction', in Elizabeth Hallam and Tim Ingold (eds), *Creativity and Cultural Improvisation*. Oxford: Berg Publishers, pp. 1–24.

Ingold, Tim, and Jo Vergunst. 2008. *Ways of Walking: Ethnography and Practice on Foot*. London: Routledge.

Jackson, Eileen. 1997. 'Dimensions of Care in Five United States Nursing Homes: Identifying Invisible Work in Care-Giving', *International Journal of Nursing Studies* 34: 192–200.

Jackson, Michael. 1995. *At Home in the World*. Durham, NC: Duke University Press.

———. 2002. *The Politics of Storytelling: Violence, Transgression, and Intersubjectivity*. Copenhagen: Museum Tusculanum Press.

Kass, Leon. 1994. *The Hungry Soul: Eating and the Perfecting of Our Nature*. Chicago: University of Chicago Press.

Kaufman, Sharon R. 1994a. 'Old Age, Disease, and the Discourse on Risk: Geriatric Assessment in U.S. Health Care', *Medical Anthropology Quarterly* 8: 430–47.

———. 1994b. 'The Social Construction of Frailty: An Anthropological Perspective', *Journal of Aging Studies* 8: 45–58.

Kayser-Jones, Jeanie Schmit. 1981. *Old, Alone, and Neglected: Care of the Aged in the United States and Scotland*. Berkeley, CA: University of California Press.

———. 2003. 'The Treatment of Acute Illness in Nursing Homes: The Environmental Context of Decision Making', in Philip Stafford (ed.), *Gray Areas: Ethnographic Encounters with Nursing Home Culture*. Santa Fe, NM: School of American Research Press, pp. 23–68.

Kearl, Michael. 1996. 'Dying Well: The Unspoken Dimension of Aging Well', *American Behavioral Scientist* 39: 336–60.

Kehoe, Mary. 1998. 'The Benevolent Asylum', *Hotham History Project*. Retrieved 14 August 2020 from https://www.hothamhistory.org.au/the-benevolent-asylum/.

Kitwood, Tom. 1993. 'Person and Process in Dementia', *International Journal of Geriatric Psychiatry* 8: 541–45.

———. 1997. *Dementia Reconsidered: The Person Comes First*. Buckingham & Philadelphia: Open University Press.

Kleinman, Arthur. 2009. 'Caregiving: The Odyssey of Becoming More Human', *The Lancet* 373: 292–93.

Laird, Carobeth. 1979. *Limbo*. Novato, CA: Chandler & Sharp.

Latimer, Joanna, and Rolland Munro. 2009. 'Keeping & Dwelling: Relational Extension, the Idea of Home, and Otherness', *Space and Culture* 12: 317–31.

Latour, Bruno. 2004. 'How to Talk about the Body? The Normative Dimension of Science Studies', *Body & Society* 10(2–3): 205–29.

Lee, Diana T.F., Jean Woo and Ann E. Mackenzie. 2002. 'The Cultural Context of Adjusting to Nursing Home Life: Chinese Elders' Perspectives', *The Gerontologist* 42: 667–75.

Lock, Margaret. 2013. *The Alzheimer Conundrum: Entanglements of Dementia and Aging*. New Jersey: Princeton University Press.

Loret, C. 2015. 'Using Sensory Properties of Food to Trigger Swallowing: A Review', *Critical Reviews in Food Science and Nutrition* 55: 140–45.

Lovatt, Melanie. 2018. 'Becoming at Home in Residential Care for Older People: A Material Culture Perspective', *Sociology of Health & Illness* 40: 366–78.

Lyon, Margaret L., and J.M. Barbalet. 1994. 'Society's Body: Emotion and the "Somatization" of Social Theory', in Thomas Csordas (ed.), *Embodiment and Experience: The Existential Ground of Culture and Self*. Cambridge: Cambridge University Press, pp. 48–66.

Mallett, Shelley. 2004. 'Understanding Home: A Critical Review of the Literature', *The Sociological Review* 52: 62–89.

Martin, Aryn, Natasha Myers and Ana Viseu. 2015. 'The Politics of Care in Technoscience', *Social Studies of Science* 45: 625–41.

McNamara, Beverley. 2001. *Fragile Lives: Death, Dying and Care*. Sydney: Allen & Unwin.

Merleau-Ponty, Maurice. 1962. *Phenomenology of Perception*. London & New York: Routledge.

Milte, Rachel, et al. 2017. 'Struggling to Maintain Individuality – Describing the Experience of Food in Nursing Homes for People with Dementia', *Archives of Gerontology and Geriatrics* 72: 52–58.

Minney, Melissa J., and Rob Ranzijn. 2015. '"We Had a Beautiful Home ... But I Think I'm Happier Here": A Good or Better Life in Residential Aged Care', *The Gerontologist* 56: 919–27.

Mol, Annemarie, Ingunn Moser and Jeannette Pols. 2010. *Care in Practice: On Tinkering in Clinics, Homes and Farms*. New York: Columbia University Press.

Musolino, Connie M. 2016. 'Assemblages of Care: Why Women with Disordered Eating are Ambivalent to Seek Therapeutic Care', Ph.D. dissertation. The University of Adelaide.

Musolino, Connie, Megan Warin and Peter Gilchrist. 2018. 'Positioning Relapse and Recovery through a Cultural Lens of Desire: A South Australian Case Study of Disordered Eating', *Transcultural Psychiatry* 55: 534–50.

Neil, Megan. 2019. 'Malnourished Aged Care Residents "Starving to Death" Warn Experts', *The Senior*. Retrieved 14 May 2020 from https://www.thesenior.com.au/story/6278038/malnutrition-a-silent-abuser-in-aged-care/?cs=13891.

Nolan, Mike, et al. 1996. 'Entry to Care: Positive Choice or Fait Accompli? Developing a More Proactive Nursing Response to the Needs of Older People and Their Carers', *Journal of Advanced Nursing* 24: 265–74.

Ouellet, Louiselle L. and Kathy L. Rush. 1996. 'A Study of Nurses' Perceptions of Client Mobility', *Western Journal of Nursing Research* 18: 565–79.

Pagone, Tony, and Lynelle Briggs. 2021. 'Care, Dignity and Respect'. Canberra, Australia: Royal Commission into Aged Care Quality and Safety.

Papadopoulos, Dimitris, Niamh Stephenson and Vassilis Tsianos. 2008. *Escape Routes: Control and Subversion in the 21st Century*. Pluto Press.

Parfit, Derek. 1984. *Reasons and Persons*. Oxford: Oxford University Press.

Parker, R.A. 1987. *The Elderly and Residential Care, Australian Lessons for Britain*. Aldershot, Hampshire, UK: Gower.

Perkinson, Margaret A. 2003. 'Defining Family Relationships in a Nursing Home Setting', in Philip Stafford (ed.), *Gray Areas: Ethnographic Encounters with Nursing Home Culture*. Santa Fe, NM: School of American Research Press, pp. 235–62.

Polanyi, Michael. 1958. *Personal Knowledge: Towards a Post-critical Philosophy*. Chicago: University of Chicago Press.

Productivity Commission. 2011a. 'Caring for Older Australians: Overview'. Canberra Productivity Commission.

———. 2011b. 'Caring for Older Australians: Volume 1'. Canberra: Productivity Commission.

Puig de la Bellacasa, Maria. 2011. 'Matters of Care in Technoscience: Assembling Neglected Things', *Social Studies of Science* 41: 85–106.

Queensland Department of Health. 2019. 'Choking'. Retrieved 4 Jan 2022 from http://conditions.health.qld.gov.au/HealthCondition/condition/1/87/257/Choking.

Rapport, Nigel. 2018. 'The Action and Inaction of Care: Care and the Personal Preserve', *The Australian Journal of Anthropology* 29: 250–57.

Rapport, Nigel, and Andrew Dawson. 1998. *Migrants of Identity: Perceptions of Home in a World of Movement*. Oxford: Berg Publishers.

Reid, Natasha, et al. 2013. 'Objectively Measured Activity Patterns among Adults in Residential Aged Care', *International Journal of Environmental Research and Public Health* 10: 6783–98.

Riebe, Deborah, et al. 2009. 'The Relationship between Obesity, Physical Activity, and Physical Function in Older Adults', *Journal of Aging and Health* 21: 1159.

Roelofs, Karin. 2017. 'Freeze for Action: Neurobiological Mechanisms in Animal and Human Freezing', *Philosophical Transactions of the Royal Society B: Biological Sciences* 372.

Rowles, Graham. 1993. 'Evolving Images of Place in Aging and Aging in Place', *Generations* 17: 65–70.

Rowles, Graham, and D. High. 2003. 'Family Involvement in Nursing Home Facilities: A Decision-Making Perspective', in Philip Stafford (ed.), *Gray Areas: Ethnographic Encounters with Nursing Home Culture*. Santa Fe, NM: School of American Research Press, pp. 173–201.

Royal Commission into Aged Care Quality and Safety. 2019. 'Royal Commission into Aged Care Quality and Safety Sydney Hearing 17 May 2019 Transcript', *Royal Commission into Aged Care Quality and Safety*.

Salmon, Eric, et al. 2005. 'Two Aspects of Impaired Consciousness in Alzheimer's Disease', *Progress in Brain Research* 150: 287–98.

Sandvoll, Anne, Kjell Kristoffersen and Solveig Hauge. 2012. 'New Quality Regulations versus Established Nursing Home Practice: A Qualitative Study', *BMC Nursing* 11: 1–7.

Savishinsky, Joel S. 2003. '"Bread and Butter" Issues: Food, Conflict, and Control in a Nursing Home', in Philip Stafford (ed.), *Gray Areas: Ethnographic Encounters with Nursing Home Culture*. Santa Fe, NM: School of American Research Press, pp. 103–20.

Sellers, Marg, and Eileen Honan. 2007. 'Putting Rhizomes to Work: (E)merging Methodologies', *NZ Research in Early Childhood Education Journal* 10: 145–54.

Sheets-Johnstone, Maxine. 2011. 'The Imaginative Consciousness of Movement: Linear Quality, Kinaesthesia, Language and Life', in Tim Ingold (ed.), *Redrawing Anthropology: Materials, Movements, Lines*. Ashgate, Farnham, UK: University of Aberdeen, pp. 115–28.

Smith, Daniel. 2018. 'What Is the Body without Organs? Machine and Organism in Deleuze and Guattari', *Continental Philosophy Review* 51: 95–110.

Somerville, Peter. 1992. 'Homelessness and the Meaning of Home: Rooflessness or Rootlessness?', *International Journal of Urban and Regional Research* 16: 529–39.

Stafford, Philip. 2003a. 'Introduction: The Nursing Home as Cultural Code', in Philip Stafford (ed.), *Gray Areas: Ethnographic Encounters with Nursing Home Culture*. Santa Fe, NM: School of American Research Press, pp. 3–22.

———. 2003b. 'Homebodies: Voices of Place in a North American Community', in Philip Stafford (ed.), *Gray Areas: Ethnographic Encounters with Nursing Home Culture*. Santa Fe, NM: School of American Research Press, pp. 121–51.

Taylor, Jenelle. 2008. 'On Recognition, Caring, and Dementia', *Medical Anthropology Quarterly* 22: 313–35.

The Senate Community Affairs Committee Secretariat. 2018. 'Effectiveness of the Aged Care Quality Assessment and Accreditation Framework for Protecting Residents from Abuse and Poor Practices, and Ensuring Proper Clinical and Medical Care Standards are Maintained and Practised'. Canberra, Australia: The Senate Community Affairs References Committee.

The Sydney Morning Herald. 1860. 'The Benevolent Asylum at New South Wales', *The Sydney Morning Herald (NSW: 1842–1954)*, 3 January 1860.

Vesperi, Maria D. 1983. 'The Reluctant Consumer: Nursing Home Residents in the Post-Bergman Rea', in Jay Sokolosovsky (ed.), *Growing Old in Different Societies: Cross Cultural Perspectives*. Belmont, CA: Wadsworth Press, pp. 225–37.

———. 2003. 'A Use of Irony in Contemporary Ethnographic Narrative', in Philip Stafford (ed.), *Gray Areas: Ethnographic Encounters with Nursing Home Culture*. Santa Fe, NM: School of American Research Press, pp. 69–102.

Warnock, Carly. 2013. 'Barefoot Running: Feeling the World through Your Feet', Master's dissertation, University of Ottawa.

Whitehead, Graham J. 2018. 'The Melbourne Benevolent Asylum Comes to Cheltenham'. Retrieved 15 December 2017 from http://localhistory.kingston.vic.gov.au/htm/article/302.htm.

Yun-Hee, Jeon, et al. 2013. 'Care Planning Practices for Behavioural and Psychological Symptoms of Dementia in Residential Aged Care: A Pilot of an Education Toolkit Informed by the Aged Care Funding Instrument', *Contemporary Nurse: A Journal for the Australian Nursing Profession* 44: 156–69.

Zerubavel, Eviatar. 1979. *Patterns of Time in Hospital Life: A Sociological Perspective*. Chicago: University of Chicago Press.

# INDEX


**A**

Activities of Daily Living (ADLs), 6, 51, 89–90, 92, 94–95
Adelaide, South Australia, 20, 41, 88, 104
affective engagement, 8, 85
ageing, 2–3, 16–19, 32
  biomedical framing of, 9–11
Alzheimer's disease, 9
  experience of, 50–51, 104, 116, 136–37
  Lock, Margaret on, 10
  Taylor, Janelle on, 59, 136–37
assemblage, 20, 45, 53
  of care, 56, 63, 71, 75, 81, 83, 98, 100–103, 112, 132
  *See also* right (assemblage of) care
assistance, 2–3, 6, 8, 13, 16, 24–25, 36, 93, 96, 105, 131
  physical, 36, 90
  *See also* staff assistance
at home, 1–5, 20
  Jackson, Michael on, 18–19
  in the nursing home, 34, 38–40, 44–45, 55–56, 70–74, 87–88, 92, 106–7, 116, 133–37
  Lovatt, Melanie on, 14–15
attention, 29, 32–34, 49, 104, 111, 113, 135–36
  conscious, 31, 34, 37–38, 69, 128–29
  instrumental, 32, 56
  lack of, 98, 105
  staff, 76, 90, 99, 105–6, 109–10
autonomy, 3, 11–13, 19, 42, 44, 49–50, 106–7, 110–11, 114–15, 133

**B**

balance: aid, 6
  between acting and being acted upon, 18–19, 49–50
  care as a, 19, 42–45, 100, 114–15
  impaired, 2–4, 29, 33, 72, 77, 79, 83, 101, 104
  improved, 34–39, 109–10
Barbaras, Renaud, 18, 32
becoming-at-home
  through movement, 12, 19–20
  in the nursing home, 110
  in walking, 40–42
behavioural and psychological symptoms of dementia (BPSD), 11
  agitation, 64–65, 104–6, 110, 121
  apathy, 66–67, 104–5, 125
  wandering, 48–49, 56–59, 134
bodies
  as assemblages, 53
  as multiplicities, 36
  synthesis, 32–33, 53–54, 68, 109–10

**C**

Care: aged, 3–4
  as assemblages, 6–7, 68–71, 94, 98–103
  duty of, 100, 106–7
  ethics of, 11–12, 42–44, 49–50, 107
  Ingold, Tim on, xi–xii
  Mol, Annemarie on, 8, 19, 81
  as multiplicities, 19, 43–45, 87, 94–97, 100–103
  as work or task, 5–6, 85–86, 99–100
care needs, 88–89, 90, 94, 100–102, 105; complex, 92–93
choice, 4, 12, 16, 19, 110–11, 114–15, 125–26, 131
control, 4, 12, 18–19, 33–34, 45, 54–56, 67, 74–75, 109–10, 133n
  loss of, 34, 40, 47–49, 64–66, 78–79, 95–96

sense of, 13–14, 39–43, 53, 79–81
taking, 43–44, 114–15, 124–25

**D**

Deleuze, Gilles
on assemblage, 6–7, 20
on becoming and desiring-production, 19–20, 65–66, 119, 130
and Guattari, Félix
on line of flight, 130
on multiplicity, 19–20, 87, 122
dementia, 12, 47, 58, 79, 104, 127
as brain pathology, 48–49, 134–35
biomedical construction of, 9–10, 48–49, 79
as a loss, 9–11, 47–49
people with, 12, 54, 57, 134–37
in residential aged care, 10–11, 26
residents with, 56–59, 106, 115, 124, 129, 136
unit, 10–11, 26, 46–48, 125
dementia care
Cohen, Lawrence on, 10
disease-centred, 10–11, 134
Kitwood, Tom on, 134–35
person-centred, 134–37
dementia with Lewy bodies, 76, 78–80, 134
Dennis, Simone, 8, 17–18
desire, 57, 63, 65, 118–19, 127
movements of, 119, 122
productive, 20, 115–16, 122, 129–30
diet, 91, 126
modified texture, 123
vitaminized, 121, 131
disability, 6, 9, 12, 36, 135

**E**

eating, 117
affected by antipsychotic medication, 120–21, 126–28
as an assemblage, 7
as multiplicities, 122, 130–31
and not eating, 114–16, 119–20, 130
as multisensory processes of, 127–28
environment, 44, 53, 55–56, 63, 79, 81, 87, 121
home-like, xxvi, 14
institutional, 98–100
nursing home, 2–4, 14–17, 24, 40, 59, 128
experience
of dying, 132; of eating, 128, 130–31
lived, 11, 13–14, 16, 17, 18, 134
of pain, 33, 92
of walking, 32, 59, 66

**F**

fall prevention
measure and strategy, 103
plan, 112
*See also* risk: fall
family, 1–3, 13, 21, 51, 63, 65, 87, 88, 90, 105, 109, 115, 117, 123, 132
feeding, 48, 86, 89, 116–19, 123–25, 127–30, 133n
fieldwork, 2, 11, 14, 19–27, 60–61, 85, 94, 96, 104, 123, 127, 131–32, 135
food, 6, 7, 91, 93
choice, 123, 131
as 'desiring-machine', 118–19
refusal, 114–15, 123–27
sensory properties of, 118, 129
texture-modified, 115–16, 121–23, 130–32
funding, 8, 82, 100–103, 112
Aged Care Funding Instrument (ACFI), 88–89, 91–94
*See also* policy: funding

**H**

habit, 40–41, 54, 58, 72, 90–91, 94–96, 108
Dewey, John on, 41
Ingold, Tim on, xi, 45
home: notion of, 12–13, 18–19, 42
sense of, 7, 13–14, 16–17, 29, 38, 42–43, 102–3, 119
taste of, 116–20

**I**

impairment, 29, 78–79, 102–3
bodily, 8, 27, 35, 61–62, 69, 81, 110, 111, 137
cognitive, 12, 16–17, 19, 20–21, 26, 47, 49, 51–59, 75, 79, 83, 94–95, 110, 115
physical, 19, 44, 69

Ingold, Tim
  on attunement or synergy, 38
  on being alive as moving through the world, 18, 52–53
  on being observant to the world, 52–53, 54
  on correspondence, 18
  on habit, 44–45
  on mind-brain, machine- or tree-body, xi
Ingold, Tim and Vergunst, Jo, 29, 53
inhabiting, 24, 40–41, 58–59, 79

**J**

Jackson, Michael, 18–19, 38, 42

**L**

life, 2–3, 29, 52, 54, 127, 132, 135
  course, 16, 49, 114
  and death: choice and control over, 114–15
  end of, 88–89, 114–15, 132–33
  everyday, 51, 76, 77, 108, 109
  nursing home, 1, 13, 91
  quality of, 2, 106, 134
  stages of, 16, 21, 29, 49, 117, 120
  threshold between, 132–33
lifeworld, 61, 79, 86
loss, 11, 13–15, 40, 50, 55, 134
  of capacity, 9, 35
  of mind and self, 10, 47–49
  of movement, 63

**M**

malnutrition, 126, 131
mealtimes, 95, 96, 132
medication, 4, 7, 47, 90, 104, 114
  antipsychotic, 103–4, 106–8, 116, 120–21, 126–28
  pain, 132
  Parkinson's, 67–68, 101
  schedule or regime, 8, 67, 71, 95–96
Merleau-Ponty, Maurice, 17–18
mind, x, 10, 19, 49, 53, 58, 126
  and body, 60, 81
  fission of, 67–68
mobility, 35. *See* movement: capability
  aid, 16–17, 103 (*see also* walking aid, frame or walker)
  assessment, 64, 91
  care, 35, 70–71, 91–92, 101–2, 106–12
  impaired, 77–81
Mol, Annemarie, 8, 19, 81
movement
  biomedical and clinical conceptualizations of, 48–49, 63, 110–11
  daily, 2, 17
  capability, 3
  concerted, 33–34, 53, 62–63
  control, 39–40, 47
  flow of movement, 31–33, 45, 56, 65–66, 73, 102–3, 116
  (in)voluntary movement, 7, 64–66, 103, 109–10
  spontaneous movement, 82, 112–13

**N**

nursing home
  as contested cultural space, 12–13, 85–86
  residents: dying, 132–33; frailty of, 9, 19; malnutrition of, 114, 126, 131–32
  staff: personal care workers (carers), 7, 36, 86, 99–100, 127; physiotherapist, 8, 24–25, 34–35, 90, 91, 92; registered nurse, 46, 47, 48, 92, 93, 101, 125
  staffing level, 113n3
nutrition, 48, 100, 117, 118–19; care, 115–16, 124

**P**

pain
  assessment, 92
  experience of, 17–18, 31–34, 67–68, 86, 91–92, 104, 126
  management plan, 92–93, 132
Parkinson's disease, 63–65
  frozen gait of, 62–63, 68–70
  medication, and 'on-and-off' phenomenon of, 67–68
personhood
  cognitive-centred, 10–11, 134
  relational-centred, 134
place, xi, 1, 3, 12–13, 18, 38, 41, 44, 47, 53, 59, 60, 70
  right, 5, 80
Polanyi, Michael, 31–33, 56, 69–70

policy
aged care, 3, 4, 11
dysphagia management, 116, 131–32
funding, 7, 8, 87, 100
restraint, 103, 108
power
of biomedical framing, 10–11
examining care through themes of, 8, 19
relations, 24–26, 86
process, 3, 24, 35–36, 40–41, 45, 52–53, 75, 91, 116
ageing, 9
of becoming, 15–16, 20, 74
of desiring-production, 19–20, 68, 119
of dying, 132
of eating, 121, 130
of walking, 54, 58
productive desire, 115–16, 122, 129–30

**R**

Rapport, Nigel
on elderly people's starving to death, 114–15
on personal preserve, 49–50
on social ethics of care, 11, 42, 43–44, 49–50, 114–15
residential aged care
as home, 2–3
as industry, 20
as medicine, 91, 87
in Australia: current crisis, 5–6, 106–7, 113n3, 123, 126; levels and types, 3, 88–89
residential aged care facility, 14, 20–24. *See* nursing home
residential aged care practice
care needs assessment, 86, 88–92, 101–2, 105, 108
care planning, 44–45, 86–87, 90–94, 100–103, 111–13
personal care, 7–8, 25–26, 85–86, 113n, 131–32
routine care, 42–43, 91, 94–97, 112–13
restraint
chemical, 103–4, 108
in nursing homes, 104, 134
physical, 103, 106; policy on, 103, 108
right (assemblage of) care, 4–5, 8–9, 19, 81–82, 92–93, 98–99, 102–3, 107–8, 111–13, 116, 131–33, 137
risk
choking, 121, 130–31
discourse of, 101–3, 106, 112
fall, 34, 99–102, 106–7 (*see* fall prevention)
malnutrition, 131
and safety, 106
routine, 129, 132. *See also* residential aged care practice: routine care
activity, 17, 41, 43, 87
institutional, 42–43, 95–97, 112
lunch, 121, 131
personal, 40, 44, 94, 96
practice, 13, 18, 41–43
staff, 96
temporal structure of, 71, 111
walking, 8, 33–34, 36, 38–45, 53–54, 62, 67–68, 70–71, 101–2
Royal Commission into Aged Care Quality and Safety in Australia, 5–6, 106–7, 113n3, 123

**S**

Savishinsky, Joel
on feeding and meanings of food, 119, 133n
on residents' rejection of food, 125
on residents' starving to death, 123
sense, 3, 5, 6, 12–16, 40, 51, 53–54, 70, 79, 90, 100, 132
of being-at-home, 4, 11, 29, 42, 45, 49
of belonging, 18, 43, 70
of control, 14, 42–43, 80–81
of home, 7, 13–14, 16–17, 19, 29, 38, 42–43, 59, 79, 102–3, 110–11, 119
of peace, 15, 34, 132
of rightness, 4, 18, 80, 102–3, 136
sitting
down, 48, 73, 76–77, 108,
prolonged, 66, 104–5
to standing, 66, 75, 76, 90, 92
up, 75, 77, 128
staff assistance, 7, 44, 51, 77, 80–81, 90–92, 94, 97, 100–2, 111–12, 124, 128
absence of, 96; insufficient, 115
prompt, 111–12
Stafford, Philip, xix, xxii, xxvii, 11, 12, 91

**T**
taste, 118–19, 122, 124, 126, 129; of home, 116–19
technology (assistive technology), 6–7, 12, 37, 81, 87, 89, 113, 115
  adjustable furniture, 4, 6–7, 108–10, 113
  call-bell system, 6–7, 96–97
  comfort (princess) chair, 7, 72–73, 80, 104, 108–9, 116, 128
  modified eating and drinking utensils, 118–19
  sensor mat system, 6–7, 82–83, 85–86, 91–92, 101–3, 111–12
tension: embodied, 27, 106
  being autonomous and being controlled by others, 11–12, 42–43, 49–50
  between care needs and care provision, 99–100, 102, 112–13
  between multiple forces, 87, 94, 97–98
  eating and not eating, 120, 130
  home and nursing home, 13–14
  policy and practice, 7, 87
  walking and not walking, 19, 29, 63–69, 72–77, 81
threshold
  between eating and not eating, 115–16, 130–32
  life and death, 114, 127, 132–33
time
  management, 96, 112
  staff, 8, 48, 93, 100–101
transfer (changing position from sitting to standing), 6, 24–26, 36, 44, 66–67, 75–77, 79–80, 85, 89–92, 94–95

**W**
walking, 29; 31–32, 53, 60–61, 89, 97–98
  and not walking: tension between, 72–75, 81
  aid, frame or walker, 1–2, 6, 36–38, 91, 95, 97–98
  as ambulation, 35, 90–91
  as an assemblage, 7–8, 45
  habit of, 58, 98
  routine, 8, 33–34, 36, 38–45, 53–54, 62, 67–68, 70–71, 101–2; staff-assisted, 8, 24, 68, 70–71, 102–3
  with care, 39–40
wandering. *See also* behavioural and psychological symptoms of dementia (BPSD)
  biomedical conceptualization, 48–51, 54–59, 134
  experience of, 46–47, 53–56, 58–61, 136–37

www.ingramcontent.com/pod-product-compliance
Ingram Content Group UK Ltd.
Pitfield, Milton Keynes, MK11 3LW, UK
UKHW021839100926
8556IPUK00004B/437